# Hypnosis to F*ck Anxiety & Stress

## Become A Superwoman with 99+ Techniques to Overcome Anxiety, Depression and Insecurity in Relationships. Guided Meditation to Quit Smoking & Drinking from Stress.

## Jackie Parks

Table of Contents

# Introduction

Anxiety is a natural response to fear or danger and can keep people safe in certain situations. Some people, however, experience anxiety more severely than others. This can lead to anxiety disorders, which can cause people to make major changes in their lives and habits to avoid situations or places that they believe cause them anxiety. If symptoms are persistent, a person might even be diagnosed with an anxiety disorder and recommended to seek treatment. Anxiety disorders can present themselves in a variety of ways; panic attacks, social anxiety, phobias, and separation anxiety to name a few.

A person might experience a host of physical symptoms with their anxiety, which can sometimes make it seem worse. Besides the unhealthy negative thoughts that are racing through their brain, they might also feel their heart racing, their temperature rising, or their breathing becoming shallower. These are all typical fight-or-flight responses that are triggered by anxiety to encourage a person to avoid the situation because the brain is perceiving it as a threat. It can be difficult for people to ignore thoughts of fear and dread when their body is pitching in and seemingly confirming them.

People experience anxiety for many different reasons, usually depending on their own life experiences and how their past has affected them. Some people have triggers for their anxiety, such as social situations or being separated from somewhere they feel is a safe space. Others feel anxiety in relation to nothing in particular but are constantly plagued with thoughts of fear and danger throughout the day. It can be difficult to deal with anxious feelings on a daily basis, but there are some things people can do to help ease the tension.

## Anxiety Explained

Anxiety can be difficult for people to recognize when they are first experiencing it. Most people, in fact, might mistake it for a physical health problem due to the symptoms that accompany it. At its core, anxiety is a response to stress. It makes people feel scared or worried about certain situations for a variety of reasons. Some people might be worried that others will judge them for how they act or speak, others might be afraid that some harm will come to them if they put themselves in a certain situation. These feelings are not all abnormal, however. Some common anxiety-inducing situations include a child's first day of school, an initial job interview, or someone's wedding day. These experiences can all cause anxiety due to the uncertainty of the situation and might cause a person to start thinking about worst-case scenarios.

All of these feelings are part of anxiety because it was the evolutionary way of keeping people safe when their environment was inherently dangerous. The heightening of senses and increased heart rate prepares the body to run or fight if presented with danger, which could have meant life or death in prehistoric times. Today, however, people are not faced with imminent death on a daily basis, but their brain might not know how to adjust itself to the safety of modern life. It can still trigger anxious feelings if it is threatened to encourage a person to flee the situation, even if the reasons are not rational.

Some people experience anxiety to an extreme degree and can feel like their negative thoughts are unrelenting. For someone with this level of anxiety, quieting their mind and finding any kind of relief can be especially difficult and might even seem impossible. If a person suffers from anxiety of this intensity for an extended period of time, they might fit the criteria for an anxiety disorder. Typically, to qualify for a disorder diagnosis, a person has to experience symptoms for longer than six months or the symptoms need to be interfering with their daily life.

There are a variety of anxiety disorders that are all defined by how the anxiety affects someone or what causes anxious feelings. Each person is different, even though they might experience similar symptoms of anxiety, and the way their anxiety affects them can make a big difference in a diagnosis. Among these disorders is a plethora of negative side effects caused by the increased levels of stress and constant negative thoughts. Some people have trouble sleeping at night, have trouble concentrating during the day, find interacting with others especially difficult, or are too afraid to leave their own homes.

Some common anxiety disorders include panic disorder, phobias, social anxiety disorder, and separation anxiety. Obsessive-compulsive disorder is no longer considered an anxiety disorder, but people diagnosed with it often experience severe anxiety as one of their symptoms. Each of these common disorders associate anxiety with a particular object, situation, or action. These disorders can severely affect a person's life by making them unable to perform daily tasks or prevent them from enjoying their hobbies. For example, someone with agoraphobia—fear of crowds—may become so debilitated by fear that they refuse to leave their home.

The symptoms of anxiety are not necessarily universal and can vary greatly from person to person. Sometimes the reason a person has anxiety can determine their symptoms, as well. For example, someone who has anxiety because they think they are in danger might feel a pounding heart because their body wants to escape. Another person, however, who is dreading a social interaction, might experience an upset stomach due to the increased stress. Symptoms can range from gastrointestinal issues to cardiovascular discomfort, headaches, and in extreme cases even vomiting if stress builds up enough with the anxiety.

At the onset of symptoms, some people may suddenly feel like they are no longer in control of their body. This can often increase feelings of anxiety because they may not feel like the dread or physical symptoms will ever subside. Sometimes this out of control feeling can even lead to panic attacks. Other startling symptoms can include nightmares or constantly recalling painful thoughts or memories. These can also contribute to increased stress and anxiety because a person might feel like they cannot escape their own negative thoughts or what might seem to be an inevitably painful outcome of an event.

In people with generalized anxiety, it is more common to worry about things because of a past experience. For example, if a child's parent forgot them in a grocery store for an extended time, that child might then develop a fear of grocery stores and feel unsafe when they go to one. This could potentially carry on into adulthood, even if the person doesn't remember the event that instigated their anxiety. Common symptoms of this type of anxiety usually present themselves when a person is in a certain situation or sometimes if they merely consider putting themselves in the trigger situation. These people often experience a racing heart, shortness of breath or rapid breathing, restlessness, trouble focusing, and a slew of other symptoms.

Anxiety can even affect a person's stomach function, causing gas, constipation, or diarrhea when it flares up. This can also contribute to more severe anxiety in a person because they may become fixated on their stomach problems and convinced that if they are in a social situation, they might have a problem they cannot get away to handle. Some people can experience this discomfort even at the thought of doing something that gives them anxiety. This is why it can be particularly difficult for people to overcome their anxiety. If even the thought of doing something makes them feel physically ill, it can be difficult to convince themselves that actually doing it won't be painful.

When people experience these intense physical symptoms in relation to their anxiety, it can often cause them to start avoiding things, situations, or people that they believe will trigger their negative feelings. Although this might seem like an effective coping mechanism to those with anxiety, it can actually severely limit their lives by making them unable to participate in normal everyday tasks. On top of wanting to avoid these situations, anxiety can make a person feel too weak or fatigued to engage in social activities. This further cements their desire to withdraw and stay confined to their safe space instead of facing and managing their anxiety.

## Causes and treatments

Most people feel anxious at some point in their life, but there can be certain factors or triggers that cause other people to feel it more severely than normal. These can include someone's genetics, their environment, how their brain is wired, and what life experiences they've had. If a person associates something with fear, it is likely they will develop anxiety surrounding that thing. Although it is typical for people to have some sort of trigger for their anxiety, this is not true for all cases. Some people have very generalized anxiety about nothing in particular; they are simply always worried or dreading being out in the world.

For some people, one type of anxiety can cause them to develop another type of anxiety. For example, someone who has anxiety about suffering harm or getting sick might develop a germ-related obsessive-compulsive disorder as a way to ensure they will never get sick. Or, people with social anxiety disorder might eventually develop agoraphobia if they never force themselves to interact with others.

Risk factors for different types of anxiety disorders typically coexist in people who suffer with them, which demonstrates that no single experience is likely to cause someone to develop a disorder. Scientists have found that nature and nurture are strongly linked when it comes to the likelihood that someone will develop severe anxiety. Genetically, research has shown that people have about a 30 to 67 percent chance of inheriting anxiety from their parents (Carter, n.d.). Although someone's DNA might be a factor in them developing anxiety, it cannot account for all of the reasons that have developed it.

Environmental factors should also be taken into consideration when trying to find the root cause of anxiety. Parenting style can be a large factor in whether or not a person will develop anxiety. If parents are controlling of their children or if they model anxious behaviors, the child might grow up thinking these are normal behaviors they should model. This can lead to feeling anxious based on a learned behavior. Other factors such as continual stress, abuse, or loss of a loved one can also elicit a severe anxious reaction because a person may not know how to handle the situation they find themselves in.

In addition to the environment, a person's health can often cause anxiety as well. If someone is diagnosed or living with a chronic medical condition or a severe illness, it can cause an anxious reaction. One possibility is if the illness is affecting the person's hormones which can cause stress, or if their feelings of not having control are worsened by a diagnosis they cannot fix.

Some people might not realize that the choices they make daily could be contributing to their anxiety. Things such as excessive caffeine, tobacco use, and not exercising enough can all cause anxiety. Caffeine and other stimulants can increase a person's heart rate and simulate anxiety symptoms. Not exercising can lower a person's level of happy hormones and make their muscles tense or sore which can also contribute to stress. A person's personality can also determine how severe their anxiety might be. Shy people who tend to stay away from conversations and interaction might develop more severe social anxiety because they are not exposed to those situations often.

When experiencing anxiety, it can seem like there is no way out, but there are actually quite a few different ways a person can work to ease their worries, ranging from clinical to holistic approaches. What type of treatments will work depends on the person, and often, how severe their struggle is.

A few clinical ways to treat anxiety include counseling, psychotherapy, and medication. These are not the only ways a person can be medically treated, but they tend to be the most conventional routes for treating mental illness. Counseling is a type of therapy where the person is able to talk to a licensed practitioner and receive feedback and advice about their situation and how to handle their emotions. Most counselors have a master's degree in the psychology field and are licensed through their state. This type of therapy is usually considered a short-term solution for people who are struggling but not debilitated by their anxiety.

Psychotherapy is typically a more long-term solution for people whose lives are impacted by their anxiety. This type of therapy can focus on a broader range of issues and triggers such as a person's anxious patterns or behaviors and how to fix them. Cognitive behavioral therapy is often used in this type of therapy to work with the person to adjust their thoughts and behaviors.

Some people find relief once prescribed medication to help them manage their anxiety. This route is usually reserved for people who are struggling the most and having trouble calming themselves on their own. There are various types of medications such as SSRIs (selective serotonin reuptake inhibitors) and SNRIs (serotonin-norepinephrine reuptake inhibitors) that alter brain chemicals to reduce anxiety or worry.

Making changes to their lifestyle and habits can also help people with anxiety relieve some of their symptoms. This is a more natural approach to managing anxiety and can be successful for people who are dedicated to making positive life changes. Small things such as diet adjustments and increasing activity levels can reduce anxious feelings. Establishing a consistent sleep schedule is also important to help someone ensure they are getting enough rest each night. Stress fatigues the body and it may need more time to fully recuperate at night if it was taxed during the day. Making sure the body has a routine can also make someone feel safe and know what to expect from their day.

Meditation can also be a good way for people to calm their minds and ease anxiety. Taking time during the day to be still and quiet might help someone stop the constant worry they feel during the day and relax for a moment. Once they start training their body to relax, it is more likely that they can keep it up during the day. Finally, avoiding stimulants such as caffeine, sugar, and tobacco, and depressants such as alcohol can greatly improve a person's chances of overcoming their anxiety. These substances contribute to the brain's hyperactivity and can often increase feelings of anxiety.

# Chapter 1    Understanding Meditation - Starting From Its History and Benefits

Meditation practitioners swear by the practice's ability to bring about sustained positive effects into their lives. One of the first questions that come to mind when you start thinking of any subject is its origin is "Who discovered meditation?" or "What are its origins?" etc. and these are a great place to start learning about it.

## History of Meditation

Well, the exact point in history or the person who 'discovered' meditation is not known at all. The word 'meditation' comes from the Latin term 'meditatum,' which means 'to ponder.' Historians and experts believe that the practice is likely to have begun thousands of years ago, far before the birth of modern civilization.

Ancient hieroglyphs and texts that have been deciphered show that even during the hunger-gatherer times, human beings practiced some form of meditation. It is believed that these traditions and practices were passed on orally through the generations, which, perhaps, forms the foundation of modern-day meditation techniques.

The earliest records of this ancient practice are from about 1500 B.C.E in the Indian subcontinent. During these ancient times, in this region, meditation was an integral part of the Vedic and other Indian philosophies. Between the 6th and 4th centuries, B.C.E. Indian Buddhist and Chinese Taoist traditions started developing their own versions of various meditation styles. In the western part of the world, notable Greek and Middle Eastern philosophers like Philo of Alexandria, Saint Augustine, and the Desert Fathers of the Middle East also developed and practiced meditation techniques.

Although many ancient religions followed meditation, it is most closely linked with Buddhism that was founded by Siddhartha Gautama or Lord Buddha in India more than 2500 years ago. Lord Buddha inspired generations of practitioners to sit and contemplate various aspects of human life and to be mindfully aware of everything happening within and around them.

According to Buddhist teachings, meditation is one of the three pillars that need to be mastered to achieve enlightenment or spiritual awakening. The people who practiced Buddha's teachings traveled the world and learned from other teachers incorporating new techniques even as they continuously endeavored to refine their own knowledge on the subject.

Eastern philosophy and meditation techniques caught the attention of Western seekers during the colonization of Asian countries by European powers from around the 18th century onward.

However, it was not until the mid-20th century that the concept and benefits of meditation became highly popular in the western world. Students from the west traveled to the eastern part of the world to train and learn from great masters. One of the most well-known western personalities of mindfulness meditation is Dr. Jon Kabat-Zinn, who founded the Center for Mindfulness at the University of Massachusetts Medical School in 1979.

His program entitled the Mindfulness-Based Stress Reduction program is credited with spreading the benefits of meditation and mindfulness practice right across the world minus all spiritual and religious overtones. Today, meditation techniques are more focused on relaxation and stress-relieving purposes rather than on achieving 'enlightenment' thought practitioners, and experts believe that the ultimate goal of meditation is to transcend human limitations and connect with the limitless universal power.

Meditation is to the mind what fitness and physical training are to the body. Meditation works like a vitalizing tonic for our minds driving it to relax and become increasingly aware of our senses and the world around us. While relaxation, temporary stress relief, and reduced anxiety are some of the short-term benefits, research studies have demonstrated the power and vast potential of meditation for the development and growth of the human mind.

A key element to meditation is the fact that it can be practiced anytime, anywhere. Meditation comes in a variety of forms, and you can choose what is best suited for you. Additionally, there is no need for any specialized equipment or a specific place or time. All you need is a few minutes and a quiet, undisturbed place where you can practice your meditation.

## Benefits of Meditation

The benefits of meditation are numerous, and relaxation and stress-release are a part of this wide repertoire. While contemporary studies continue to try and understand the beneficial aspects of meditation on the body and mind through scientific means, it is worth mentioning here that the ultimate goal of meditation is not really to get any benefit.

Like many Eastern philosophers, meditation has no goal. It is only a tool to help you be 'in the present' and mindful of everything that is happening within and around you. According to Buddhism, the final goal of meditation is to liberate your mind from the attachment to things that you cannot control, including your own powerful emotions as well as external circumstances. This 'liberated' practitioner is then able to give up desires which result in attachment. Consequently, he or she can maintain inner harmony and lead a calm, stress-free, and meaningful life.

In the 1970s, Dr. Herbert Benson, a researcher at Harvard University Medical School, coined the phrase "relaxation response" based on studies he conducted on people who practiced meditation regularly. He defined this phrase as an involuntary response of the brain that results in reducing activity in the sympathetic nervous system, which is responsible for stress-related responses, including fight-flight reactions.

Since then, a lot of studies have been and continue to be done across the world. All of these studies have demonstrated multiple short-term benefits of meditation, especially on the functioning of the nervous system. Some of these short-term benefits of meditation are:

- Reduced blood pressure

- Improved blood circulation

- Lower and relaxed heart rate

- Reduced sweating

- Reduced cortisol levels, the stress-originating hormone

- Reduced anxiety and stress

- Increased feelings of well-being

- Improved states of relaxation

As an increasing number of people are realizing the potential benefits of meditation and this tool is slowly growing in popularity as a means of not only for temporary stress relief and relaxation but also as a supplementary therapy for multiple health disorders. Numerous research studies demonstrate the efficacy of meditation in treating diseases depression, age-related memory issues, addictions, and more. Let us look at some of the benefits that have the backing of scientific research.

**Reduces Stress** - One of the most common and useful symptoms of meditation that attracts people is its promise of stress reduction. Several studies have shown the efficacy of meditation techniques in helping people to manage stress and eliminate the negative impacts of stress on their lives.

One of the primary hormones produced in the human body that is connected with stress is cortisol, the levels of which increase with increased mental and physical stress on the body. Cytokines are inflammation-promoting chemicals whose production increases when cortisol levels are high. These harmful chemicals in the body are responsible for sleep disruption, increased blood pressure, increased anxiety, and stress - all of which contribute to reduced focus and fatigue.

Studies on mindfulness meditation have shown reduced stress-related inflammation response in the body. In fact, the higher the levels of stress in your body, the more effectively the meditation techniques work. Meditation is also believed to relieve physical symptoms of stress like post-traumatic stress disorder, irritable bowel syndrome, and fibromyalgia.

*Controls Anxiety* - When stress levels are low, anxiety levels also decrease. Meditation is known to help control symptoms of anxiety disorders that come in the form of paranoia, social anxiety, phobias, panic attacks, and obsessive-compulsive disorders. Mindfulness meditation has been found to help to reduce depression in adults.

Consistent practice has also been shown to help people manage anxiety long-term. It has also been seen to have helped in the reduction of work-related stress, especially in high-pressure environments. Nurses across the world find meditation hugely helpful in keeping their high levels of stress in check.

*Increases Self-Awareness* - Some types of meditation are designed to increase self-awareness through continuous self-inquiry. As you practice this kind of meditation and get numerous answers to questions about yourself, your self-awareness gets a big boost. Consequently, the chances of self-actualization, or being your best self, increases significantly.

Also, some forms of meditation teach you to identify and manage negative, self-defeating, and harmful thoughts. The primary aim of such kinds of meditation techniques is to help you gain an improved sense of self and more control over your thinking processes. This awareness can be used to get rid of harmful habits and inculcate useful, productive habits for an improved quality of life.

Breast cancer-afflicted women who underwent tai chi programs to handle depression issues were able to control their emotions better than the ones who did not use any kind of meditation technique as a supplementary therapy. Further, meditation helps reduce feelings of loneliness, especially among older men.

Increased self-awareness helps in improving problem-solving skills, too, both at a personal as well as a professional level. Self-awareness through meditation is the starting point of multiple positive changes in your life.

*Improves Emotional Health* - In addition to helping to manage stress and anxiety, meditation is also known to aid in improving emotional health. When you meditate regularly, your self-awareness increases significantly, which has a direct positive impact on your self-image and in having a more positive outlook on life.

The persistent practice of regular meditation helps to reduce depression in the long-term. Scientists opine that this reduced level of depression is directly related to reduced production of cytokines, which are inflammatory chemicals produced in the body in response to stress and anxiety, which leads to depression.

Comparative studies were conducted on the brain activities of people who meditate and those who did not. These studies showed considerable, measurable changes in brain activity in regular meditators, especially in the regions connected with optimism and positive thinking.

*Improves Focus and Attention Span* - Problems with focus, attention span, and concentration are not just for kids. These problems affect a multitude of adults around the world, regardless of being diagnosed with attention deficiency disorder (ADD) or not.

Just like how muscle-building and endurance exercises strengthen your muscles, meditation facilitates the strengthening of your focus and attention span. As you meditate regularly, your ability to reorient your wandering mind to bring back its attention to the work at hand will improve considerably.

With continued practice, you will find that you can stay focused on one particular task with increasing ease. Also, your memory will get a boost, as well. Some studies have also shown that meditation makes it possible to reverse and correct brain patterns that contribute to poor attention, excessive worrying, and wandering of the mind.

The best part is that you can feel these benefits within short periods of meditation exercises. Studies on people preparing for the Graduate Record Examination (GRE) showed that their focus and memory for the verbal reasoning section improved considerably with just two weeks of meditation practice.

*Reduces Age-Related Memory Loss* - Studies of Kirtan Kriya, a specific type of meditation in which participants chant a mantra while making repetitive finger movements to improve focus, reveal that age-related memory loss can be slowed down.

Multiple studies on the elderly showed that various types of meditation styles helped in improved mental sharpness, memory, and attention span of the participants. Also, some dementia-affected patients showed partial improvement in memory through meditation. Meditation is also useful for caregivers of elderly patients with dementia, both family members, as well as professional caregivers.

*Increases Kindness and Compassion* - Certain types of meditation like Metta or loving-kindness meditation, help develop kindness and compassion toward everyone, including yourself. Ideally, this kind of meditation starts by developing kindness toward yourself and then projecting this kindness onto other people around you.

Loving-kindness meditation helps you extend the self-compassion you develop first to friends and loved ones, then to acquaintances and strangers, and ultimately even to your enemies. Multiple surveys have shown that people who practiced meditation felt increasingly compassionate toward themselves as well as others.

Also, studies demonstrated that this feeling of kindness and compassion was directly proportional to the dose of meditation. The more you meditate on loving-kindness, the more positive feelings you will be able to generate into your life. Consistent practice of Metta meditation has also been shown to reduce social anxiety, conflicts in marriages and help with anger management.

*Improves **Quality of Sleep*** - Thanks to the stresses of modern times, a large percentage of the world's urban population is diagnosed and treated for insomnia. In studies that worked with controlled groups, it was noticed that the group who meditated reported improved quality of sleep and sleep patterns, whereas the participants who did not practice meditation continued to have sleep-related problems.

Meditation helps you fall asleep sooner and helps you sleep for a longer period. A skilled practitioner can redirect racing thoughts that are one of the primary causes of insomnia. Meditation also helps to relax your body, release tension, and takes you to a peaceful state of mind, all of which are excellent sleep triggers.

Therefore, meditation techniques are great to control and redirect runaway thoughts that hamper sleep in addition to helping you to relax and release tension in your body and mind. Consequently, the time taken to fall asleep is reduced, and you also end up getting a more restful sleep than without practicing meditation.

*Helps Fight Addictions* - Meditation calls for an immense amount of mental discipline. As you progress from a novice meditator and increase the quality and quantity of time and energy you invest in meditation, you will see your mental power and willpower strengthening slowly and steadily. The self-awareness achieved through meditation also helps to improve your self-control. All of these positive impacts are highly useful in identifying and controlling addictive behaviors.

Research studies have shown that meditation helps practitioners to redirect their attention and focus productively, teaching them better emotional control. When you practice meditation regularly, you will find it easy to identify the root cause of your addictions for which you can find ways to root out these nasty behaviors from your life.

Studies have shown that people who meditate regularly tend to have better control over their cravings and also manage their craving-related stress in a much better way than those who do not meditate. Experts opine that the reason for the potential of meditation techniques helping people overcome addiction lies in the fact that meditation helps people disconnect the act of addiction (such as drinking, smoking, binge-eating, etc.) from the state of craving. Encouraged by the results of such studies, physicians also recommend meditation as part of the treatment for recovering alcoholics.

Therefore, meditation is also known to help you control the food cravings, and that results in reduced binge and emotional eating behaviors. Meditation helps a person develop willpower and mental discipline, which in turn, helps you identify and avoid unwanted impulses and cravings that form the root cause of addictions.

*Helps with Pain Management* – Both Psychiatrists and physicians believe that pain management is more about managing your state of mind than overcoming its physical aspects through painkillers. Experts, through various studies, have concluded that the effects of pain can be elevated by stress. As such, meditation is a great way of calming and relaxing your mind and is an effective pain management tool.

Studies on the brain activity of meditation practitioners showed that there is an increased amount of activity in the areas that are known to control and manage pain. People who practice meditation also reported reduced sensitivity to pain. Even in the long-term management of chronic or intermittent pain, meditation techniques are useful as a supplementary therapy.

In all the studies conducted, non-meditating and meditating participants experienced the same causes of pain. Those who meditated demonstrated a greater ability to manage and cope with pain than those who did not meditate regularly. Therefore, experts opine that meditation has the power to reduce the perception and sensitivity to pain, which, in turn, makes it an excellent supplementary therapy for chronic and intermittent pain management.

*Helps to Reduce Blood Pressure* - Meditation is also known to reduce strain on the heart, which, in turn, helps to reduce blood pressure and other stresses related to the vascular system. High blood pressure is one of the primary causes of strain on the heart as it makes the heart work harder to pump enough blood needed by the body. This continued strain and stress on the heart can lead to reduced functionality.

Narrowing of the arteries or atherosclerosis is another harmful effect of high blood pressure, which can lead to strokes and heart attacks. Studies have shown that multiple types of meditation techniques have the potential to reduce blood pressure significantly, especially for the elderly.

Meditation is believed to relax the nerve signals coordinating heart function resulted in controlled blood pressure. These nerve signals also impact the tension in blood vessels as well as the fight-or-flight responses, both of which increase during stressful conditions.

It has been seen that meditation not only reduces blood pressure during the time of practice but also in the long-term, especially for regular practitioners. Reduced blood pressure directly decreases the strain and stress on heart functions, thereby preventing vascular and heart-related diseases.

# Chapter 2    How to Set Up a Meditation Environment

Setting up your meditation environment and preparing for meditation are very important. Of course, if you are practicing walking meditation, the world is your meditation environment, however, if you are practicing any type of seated meditation, you will have to create an environment that will allow you to get the most out of your meditation sessions.

Imagine how wonderful it would be to have a dedicated area to use for healing your mind, body and spirit. That is exactly what you are going to create when you begin setting up your meditation environment. Now don't get me wrong, you don't have to have a huge house, you don't have to dedicate an entire room to your meditation area. The truth is, even a small corner will work as long as you know how to set it up properly and that is exactly what I will be teaching you in this chapter.

The first thing that you need to understand is that there are no real rules when it comes to setting up a meditation environment. However, there are some things that you need to take into consideration, ways that you can create a loving and carefree environment that will help you reach a true state of relaxation while you are meditating.

The first thing that you need to do is find a space that makes you feel good. Many people do not want to set up their meditation area in their office because this is not an area that brings them peace. Often, the opposite is true, the home office can be a place to work and pay bills, but it is not a place that people find relaxation.

The area that you choose needs to be free from traffic and it needs to be a quiet area that is not full of distractions. The room should also have access to natural light. If you are unable to find a space in your home that fits all of these requirements, you may want to consider setting up an area on your deck or even creating a space in your garden just for meditating. If you choose to meditate outside, you need to ensure that it is an area where you will feel comfortable and free from the prying eyes of the nosy neighbors.

The next step in creating your meditation environment is to clean it up and get rid of the clutter. We all have clutter in our lives. However, you need to make sure that your meditation environment is clutter-free because it can be very distracting while you are trying to meditate. This is especially true if you are the type of person that likes a clean space.

Consider emptying everything out of the space, finding a different home for it so that when you are finished creating your meditation environment, the only items that are in the area are those that improve your ability to meditate. Even if you only use a small corner of a room, you should consider finding a different place for the items that are currently in that area and dedicating that small space just to meditate.

If your space is inside, you should also consider bringing in some outside elements. Nature helps people relax naturally; this is why many people feel best when they are close to nature. Take the curtains off of the windows, add some fresh cut flowers, sand in jars, seashells, plants or a water fountain.

A small water fountain is something that you should consider using in your meditation room because you will be able to relax to the sound of the water trickling through the fountain, and this relaxing sound will help to drown out any background noise such as the television, kids playing or traffic outside.

Now it is time for you to think about the background music that you want to listen to while you are meditating. Of course, if you are practicing guided meditation, this is not something that you will have to worry about at the moment because guided meditations already have music in the background. However, if you are practicing mindfulness meditation or other meditation techniques, you will want to consider how you want to play the music and what music will be played.

Simply purchasing a cheap CD player and a CD of classical music will provide you with the background music that you need while you are meditating. It is important for you to listen to music that does not have lyrics and that it is not music that you would listen to outside of meditating.

The reason for this is because while we all love music, it can be very distracting; you do not want your favorite pop music or hard rock music playing while you are trying to meditate because you might find you want to sing along, let alone the various thoughts the lyrics could create.

Not only is classical music going to help you meditate, but it is going to provide you with other benefits as well. Classical music has been proven to increase motivation, improve sleep, ease pain, improve a person's mood while reducing stress and improving a person's IQ.

Classical music while recommended is not required. You could instead listen to the sound of the ocean; nature sounds, such as birds chirping or any other sound that you find relaxing. You should make sure that whatever track you are listening to is going to be long enough so that you will not have to stop your session and press play or change the disc. You do not want to be interrupted while you are meditating.

You may also decide that you want to add in the element of Aromatherapy. Aromatherapy is the use of essential oils to help soothe the mind, body and soul. Essential oils such as peppermint, lavender, and chamomile are great to use while you are meditating to not only relax your mind but your body as well.

Not only are essential oils able to help you relax, but studies have shown that using essential oils has many other benefits as well, such as boosting the immune system, relieving pain and reducing stress.

Next, you will want to add a few personal touches to your meditation space. You do not want a space that does not feel like it is part of who you are or that it does not belong in your house. Instead, you want your space to be comfortable, and you want it to contain some of your personal belongings.

You should, however, make sure that you are not overcrowding the space because this will cause your mind to become overcrowded while you are trying to meditate. Instead, keep the area clear of too much clutter, keep the lines clean, and only use a few pieces at a time. Remember, you can swap them out for other pieces at a later date if you find something you want to put in your meditation area. You should not, however, continue to purchase items to place in the area without taking anything out.

You need to remember how important it is for you to have fresh air in your meditation area. Of course, Aromatherapy is beneficial, but you also need to ensure that you have access to fresh air in your meditation environment. If your meditation environment is outdoors, this will not be an issue, however, if you have a meditation space inside, it may be a bit more difficult.

If you are in a room with windows, simply opening a window and turning on a fan while you are meditating will provide you with enough fresh air. On the other hand, if your meditation area does not have any windows, you may want to consider purchasing an air purifier as well as a standing fan to ensure you are getting the fresh air that your body needs.

You should also think about the color of the paint in the area. You want colors to be calming, not bright or exciting. You have to remember that you want the colors in the room to match the mental state that you are trying to reach, in other words, you want them to be calm.

The lighting is going to make a huge difference when it comes to the meditation area. If you use a curtain, it should be made out of a sheer fabric that will allow the light in, but will also allow you some privacy. If there is no natural lighting in the room, you will need to make sure you have the proper lighting fixtures. It will be up to you to decide what type of lighting you want, whether it be bright or dim, you should choose what makes you the most comfortable and helps you to relax. You should avoid florescent lights if at all possible.

You also need to ensure that your meditation area is a no-technology-allowed space. There should be, no cell phones or any other technology, except for what you will be playing your music on or your guided meditation if that is what you are using.

If you do have to have your laptop or tablet with you to listen to music or guided meditations, you need to ensure that you are only using it for that purpose. You should never check your email, get on social media or start surfing the net instead of meditating in your meditation environment. You have the entire rest of your home to complete these tasks, don't let them interfere with your meditation space.

Some people like to light candles while they are meditating, other's find that they meditate best if they are locked in the bathroom and enjoying a bubble bath. No matter where it is that you are meditating, you need to make sure that it is an environment that is relaxing to you and will allow you to be free from all distractions during the meditation process. You also need to ensure that you will not be interrupted nor will you be rushed during your sessions.

Once you have your meditation area prepared, you need to prepare yourself for the meditation session. Before I begin talking about how you can prepare yourself for meditation, you should understand that these are not rules, these are simply some ways for you to make your meditation sessions more effective.

You do not have to use these techniques when you are preparing to meditate, in fact, you could be sitting in your office right now and meditate. You see, you can meditate anywhere and anytime. However, when you create a meditation environment, as I previously talked about, and you follow the tips that I am going to give you to help you prepare for your meditation session, you will be able to benefit even more from your sessions.

The first thing that you need to do is plan your meditation times no sooner than 1 hour after you have eaten. If you do have to eat before you meditate, you should make sure that it is a very light and healthy snack. Eating a heavy, fatty meal before you meditate is only going to make you tired, and you are not going to be able to focus on the meditation session.

Some people also prefer to shower before they meditate because it symbolizes washing and cleansing of the body. This action is of course not necessary. However, it can help prepare the mind and body for meditation and help you reach a more relaxed state.

When you are preparing to meditate, you want to make sure that you are wearing comfortable clothing. These should not be too tight, and they should ensure that you do not get too hot while you are meditating, or too cold either.

Many people love to exercise before they meditate because it helps them to relax their mind and body, preparing them for the meditative state that they are trying to find. It also helps to clear the mind, allowing the person to focus only on what they are doing, and helps the mind switch from the work day to home time. Exercising is going to help ensure your body has the oxygen that it needs, your blood is flowing properly, and that your muscles are stretched. If you do not want to exercise before you meditate, you need to make sure that you are taking a few moments to stretch your muscles, helping them to relax before you begin meditating.

You may also want to take a few minutes 'time-out' before you begin meditating just to prepare your mind for what you are about to do. It is best that you do not jump from one task to the next without taking a few moments to allow your mind to adjust to the new task.

This is important for you to remember while you are switching tasks in any area of your life, but it is very important for you to remember when you start meditating. Allowing your mind to have a few minutes between tasks is going to ensure that you are able to focus only on your meditation session and not on the task that you were taking part in before meditating.

Taking part in deep breathing exercises is a great way for you to prepare your mind and your body for a meditation session. Focusing on deep breathing for 10- 15 breaths, inhaling through the nose and out the mouth, is going to help to relax the mind and help your body transition from whatever activity you were previously doing to your meditation session.

Whatever you choose to do to prepare yourself for meditation, it should be something that you find relaxing, something that helps you take your focus off of the stress of the day and onto the process of meditation.

# Chapter 3    Meditation for Anxiety

Throughout this book, we have taken the time to understand anxiety, its triggers, signs, and some of the types of anxiety disorders. It has become clear that everyone faces anxiety at one point in their lives while others seem to have it constantly haunting them. It also became clear how the word does not get the recognition it deserves.

In this chapter, we are going to look into different meditation techniques which are used to deal with anxiety and panic disorders. If you are suffering from either, this is the book for you. Who knows, it might save you the frequent trips to the doctor to get anxiety pills. Systematically, this chapter guides the reader through the various techniques known to deal with both anxiety and panic attacks.

## Anxiety and Stress Relief

The goal of anxiety and stress relief meditation is to learn how to let go of whatever is weighing you down and realize the peace and calmness the mind can experience. It serves the purpose of helping someone understand the position they are now in. The past and the future are impermanent. By letting these thoughts cloud our judgment and state of mind, we accept the troubles they drag along with them.

When it comes to anxiety and stress relief, it is highly advisable to separate yourself from everyone else. You need time to restore yourself to your most productive element because you might rub off some of the bad energy onto others. If need be, hide in a properly ventilated closet-as long as you are comfortable.

Close your eyes and try to relax your body. This is important to prepare it to get into a state of well-being. Focus your attention on yourself. This is your time; forget all the other things that cloud your mind. You want to be at peace and resonate peace and this is your time to manifest its existence. Start by inhaling and exhaling slowly through the nose and mouth in that order. Observe your body and the buildup of tension accumulated from the anxiety and stress.

You can imagine a stream of river passing and washing away all the buildup of anxiety and stress. Let it all go; let it all wash away. You can imagine anything. You can also decide to fold your stress and anxiety in a leaf and let it go in whichever direction the wind decides. Every time you exhale, envision all the worries go away. Your mind is your palace of imagination. You can do anything in the space you have created for yourself now.

Slowly, go back and observe your breathing again. Keep inhaling through your nose and exhaling through the mouth. You can decide to let it happen naturally or give it intervals of three seconds. Your space your choice. If your mind keeps wandering, you can perform a couple of deep breaths to bring back your focus to your breathing.

Now, imagine you are all alone at the beach and you have worn your favorite pair of swimsuits. You want to take a dip because you are aware of the calming effect water has on you. Picture yourself running towards the water and splashing your way in. To your surprise, when you take a dip, you start to glow and feel so nice. The more you dip yourself into the water, the more your worries wash away leaving you with a nice aura and a sense of peace. Keep imagining this before going back to observe your breathing.

Notice if there is any change in your breathing. Does it feel more natural and relaxed? Do you feel better? If not, start with the breathing again. Center yourself and your thoughts. Do not let your source of stress or anxiety plague you in this space. Remember, this is your personal space. This is your time. Nobody can take away your time.

You can use any relevant scenario as a visual tool to let go of the stress and anxiety that had manifested itself. It does not have to be exactly what is above. If it works for you, that is all that matters. Keep transitioning from your breathing to visual scenarios until the time you desire. Even after feeling better, you might decide to continue doing it for a while just because you can. There is certainly no harm in that.

Apart from the above method, mindfulness meditation, some audio guided meditations and Vipassana meditation serve as good alternatives to try. The practice of meditation does not restrict you from trying out something different if the one you are accustomed to doing does not show results. Any technique that is good for you is the best.

## Self-Healing for On-The-Spot Anxiety

Anxiety can clock in at any time it feels like. Let us compare it to that manager who decides to walk into the office, yet nobody expected them to show up because it was their day off. From minor misunderstandings to large problems, anxiety always comes packed differently to every individual. Luckily, several methods that deal with anxiety immediately occur exist. These methods are:

## Mindful Breathing

Take some time out for yourself for just five minutes. If you cannot, just pay attention to yourself wherever you are and start to breathe deeply while assuming an upright posture. Notice how the lower section of your bells expands as you breathe in through your nose and contracts as you breathe out through your mouth. Deep breathing is associated with lowering the heart rate, which in turn reduced blood pressure.

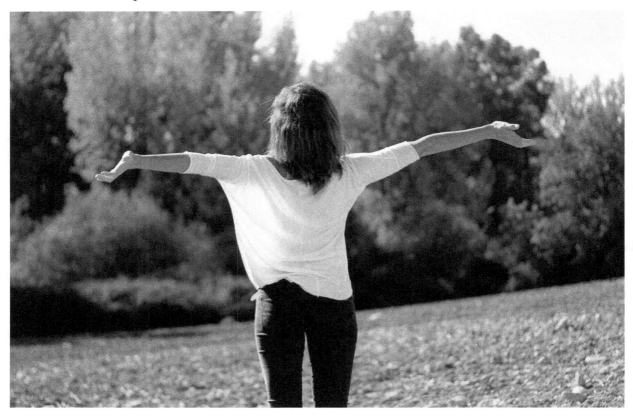

## Focus on the Present

As soon as you feel the anxiety starting to kick in, in whatever situation you are, just start to focus on what is happening presently. If you are walking, focus on how your feet hit the ground and how the wind is blowing against your face or hair. If you are eating, focus on how your fingers feel holding that spoon. What kind of sensations do you feel around your mouth as you eat? Pay attention to these details and slowly witness yourself starting to feel less tense.

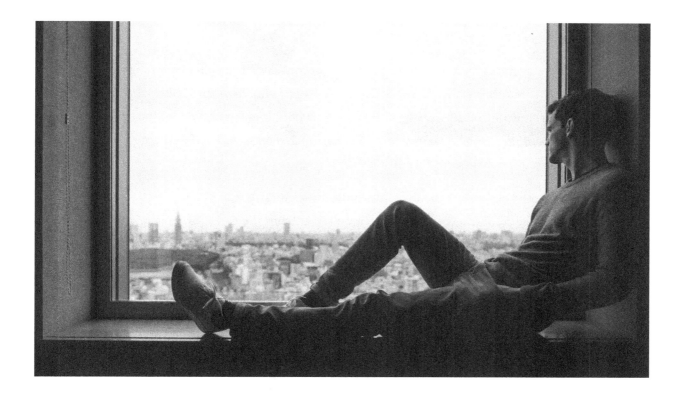

## Scan Your Body

This technique combines bodily awareness and breathing. It helps individuals experience the connection between the body and the mind. Start by observing your breathing. Inhale and exhale through your nose. The purpose is to clear all the stories in your head and concentrate on yourself. After a few minutes, focus your attention on a specific group of muscles and release any tension you feel. Move to the next muscle and so the same. Keep doing this until you have covered the whole body. You can do it in whatever order you like.

## Use Guided Imagery

Due to the availability of the internet, it is easy to find apps or audios online that can help you create guided images. However, this technique might not be so efficient for people who have a problem constructing mental images. If you have the ability to construct mental images with ease, make sure that the imageries are relatable to you. Otherwise, you might not understand what is going on-which beats the whole point. Guided imageries are there to help someone reinstate the positivity in themselves. If you find it difficult to visualize such images in your mind, you can stare at one imagine for a few seconds, and then close your eyes with the idea of retaining the image in your mind. As you practice this technique, you will find it to be easier and easier to achieve mental imagery.

## Start Counting

In school, it was a common thing to hear teachers or parents say, "If you feel angry or you want to say something out of bitterness, just count to ten first." It is funny how this holds true. Counting is one of the many easy ways to deal with your anxiety anywhere it occurs. You do not have to count to ten; you can even do it to one hundred if it feels right. Challenge yourself and count backward as well. This way, you can really get your mind into it.

Sometimes the anxiety goes away quickly, while other times it does not. Whatever the case, ensure you try to keep calm and collected. Counting distracts you from the cause of anxiety and keeps your mind busy. This will eventually return you to a state of calm.

## Interrupt Your Thoughts

From my experience with anxiety, your thoughts can so powerful to the extent of making you actually feel like your fears are going to manifest themselves. The thought itself then again doubles your anxiety and the cycle just keeps going. Then again, you realize that the majority of these things never get to happen and that you were so anxious for no good reason.

Interrupting your thoughts as they come can bring you back to a sense of calm. You can do this by starting to think about a person you love- a person who brings peace into your life. If you like a certain music album, skip to your favorite songs and jam along. Remember to always return your focus to yourself and observe how you feel after a few minutes. Observe how none of these feelings is permanent.

With these few tips, you are ready to break your anxiety cycle.

## Panic Attacks

A panic attack is an unexpected feeling of intense fear that leads to other serious physical responses where no actual risk or obvious cause is present. They may occur at any time, even when you are asleep. Sometimes they have no trigger. A panic attack gives you breathing difficulties, makes your heart pound and it gives you a feeling that you are going crazy or are about to die. It is not a pretty experience just from what it sounds like. Other symptoms that occur may include sweating, shaking, fever, nausea, your legs may 'turn to jelly' and feeling a disconnection from yourself.

Many people only get to experience less than five panic attacks in their lifetime. The problem usually then goes away after the stressful episode has ended. Some people have very constantly recurring panic attacks and they happen to stay in constant fear with the danger of having another panic attack-these people suffer from a condition called panic disorder.

It is difficult to pinpoint what exactly causes feelings of panic and the onset of attacks, but they tend to be common in families. Major life events such as marriage, graduation and retirement and the death of someone you love also show a bond with panic attacks and panic disorders. Some medical conditions can also be cause panic attacks such as hyperthyroidism and low blood sugar. The use of stimulants in the likes of caffeine and cocaine can also trigger panic attacks and disorders. If you suffer from panic disorders, it would be advisable to refrain from such.

In the event that you have had a panic attack and it has passed, it would be nice to give your body what it needs. You might feel fatigued, hungry, or even thirsty. Make sure you give yourself some good treatment after it happens. It is advisable to inform someone that you can confide in about the situation. It is not a bad thing to ask for help.

Below are breathing techniques that reverse the symptoms of panic disorders.

## Diaphragm Meditation for Panic Attacks

When we encounter a situation of distress, the pattern and rate of our breathing become different. On a normal day, we always breathe slowly using our lower lungs. However, in situations of distress, our breathing shifts to be shallow and rapid while situated in the upper lungs. In the event that it happens when resting, it can cause hyperventilation. This also explains some of the symptoms experienced during panic. Luckily, by knowing how to change your breathing, you can start to reverse the symptoms of your panic attack.

The body has a natural calming response called the parasympathetic response that triggers by changing how you breathe. It is very powerful and is the complete opposite of the emergency response (the feelings that kick in during an attack). When the calming response comes into play, all the primary changes brought about by the emergency response start to shift.

The two meditation techniques recommended to help with this disorder are natural breathing technique and the calming counting technique. The natural breathing technique is pretty much the same thing as the abdominal breathing technique. If you can practice breathing like this on a daily basis, it will only prove beneficial.

## The Natural Breathing Technique (Abdominal Breathing Method)

Gently inhale a normal amount of air through your nostrils making sure it fills your lower lungs. You can decide to place your hands beneath your lower belly to supervise this or you can do whatever seems comfortable. Make sure to exhale easily while focusing on the movements of your lower belly. Feel it expand as air gets in and go down when you exhale. Carry this practice with a relaxed mindset not forgetting to fill your lower lungs with air. Try your best to actually "feel" the oxygen rushing into your body and making its way through your blood. You will feel how every tissue in your body imbibes the fresh oxygen you have just inhaled.

## Calming Counts

Assume a comfortable sitting posture and take a deep breath. As you are exhaling, slowly whisper to yourself to relax. Keep your eyes closed to avoid losing focus. Now, start taking natural breaths while counting down from a desired number. Make sure to only count after a successful exhale. As you keep breathing, throw your attention to any areas of tension. Imagine the tension getting loose and shriveling, leaving you feeling calm and refreshed.

When you arrive at the end of your countdown, open your eyes, and notice any difference in what you are feeling. If it has worked but not as efficiently as desired, give it a longer try making sure your willpower is set to let go of the panic. Eventually, you will notice yourself get better.

Studies have shown that these meditation techniques, if practiced even when one is not anxious, are bound to yield the same results. If you can, dedicate a little time every morning and evening to practice the technique that works best for you.

Two things should be highly observed when practicing these techniques: focusing on changing negative thoughts and not thinking of anything else while meditating. This is because our thoughts directly influence our breathing and changing your negative thoughts can help lessen the symptoms quickly. Concentrate most of your effort into not thinking about anything else. Do not even think about your next breath; it should happen naturally.

# Chapter 4    Relaxation Techniques for Anxiety

When it comes to anxiety, finding the right techniques to help with relaxation is essential. That's because, if you don't have this, you won't be in control of your anxiety, and that in turn can make it harder for you to well, do something about it. But we'll talk about here the top relaxation techniques for anxiety, and how to accomplish these.

**Body Scan**

This is a type of focus that works with progressively relaxing the muscles. You'll want to make sure that your body is friendly and relaxed before you begin, but what you do for starters is you initially focus on a singular part of your body or a group of muscles all at a time. Start from your foot and begin with your toes, focusing on those.

At this point, since any of the tension that is there, and from there, start to release this tension that is sitting there mentally. You want to make sure that you do this with each side, not forgetting one over the other, and from there, star to progressively move up the body. The purpose of a body scan is used to help with awareness of the mind-body connection. If you do feel like you're out of the body in a sense, sometimes this can make you feel more grounded, and less in your head.

This is especially good for those who want to have something that will help after surgery, or something that is affecting your body image, or any issues with body image that might be bothering them. This is a good one that can help with relaxing the body too and is actually a great one to do right before bed.

**Visualization**

This is another trendy one for both stress and anxiety for various reasons. What you want to do, is first and foremost stay in a place where you can be unbothered. This can, later on, be used during a situation where you feel anxious.

What you want to do, is to imagine or picture yourself in an environment that is calming and serene. A beach with the waves hitting your feet, a small meadow filled with flowers, a place that is soothing in your head, whatever it might be, start to visualize this. Get really deep with the visualization. Actually, picture yourself standing there, and what each of your sense is feeling, and from there, start to feel your thoughts as they soothe at this point.

By merely seeing yourself in a setting that is rejuvenating and lovely, this actually allows for the body and mind to relax, and you'll feel as though you're there. It's quite amazing what this can do, and honestly, sometimes just taking five minutes out of your day to do this can make you feel like you're really there, and sometimes, this can be seen as "going to your happy place" more than anything else.

It's compelling, and it also will help you forget about the anxiety and stress.

## Self-Care Strategies

Self-care is actually something that you should also be looking at as a means to help treat stress and anxiety. When you're anxious, you're not actually working on yourself, but you need to look at activities that will help you with your health, whether it be emotional, spiritual, physical or related aspects that your personal wellness is involved with. You can look into finding different things that you should be doing, including getting enough rest, eating right, finding good social support, and also looking at your physical fitness desire, and being able to look at the different relaxation techniques can be useful when trying to include these in overall wellness and self-care as well. If you're looking to really have a means that will help you with relaxing and being better, sometimes just finding the right people can do it for you, and it will help you in life.

This can even involve some of the different soothing activities that will help you feel better. Sounds, including music that you enjoy and nature sounds and little sounds of babbling brooks and the ocean, can help some like to use aromatherapy, including incense and candles that can help. Heck, even just getting out and hiking, swimming, walking around the park, or whatever can be beneficial ways to relax.

## Progressive muscle relaxation

This kind of ties into body scan, but it's a little bit more than that. It allows you to relax different parts of your muscles. With enough practice, it will give you an intimate familiarity with the tension, and relaxation that you feel in the body. This can help with reacting to the first signs of tension that come with stress, and you'll begin to realize that as you relax, your mind does too.

The first thing that you must do talks to the doctor and find out if you've got a history of back spasms, back issues, or injuries that might be aggravated with the muscle tension. What you want to do, is work at the feet once again, and you only want to tense the muscles that you want to tense up. To begin, first you must get comfortable, take a few moments to breathe with deep breaths, and when you're ready, put the attention on the right foot, focusing on how it feels. Slowly start to tense the muscles within the right foot, squeezing this as tightly as you can for a count of about 10 or so. Relax the foot, and then focus on the tension flowing from the foot as it starts to become loose and limp and notice how it feels when you finally do take the tension off of there.

For a moment, then you want to start to focus on the relaxed state, keeping your breathing nice and slow. From there, shift towards the left foot, doing the same technique for tension and release. Move all the way up the body, going towards all of the different muscle groups. You may notice that it does take some practice at first, but once you start to get used to it, it's much more comfortable. Don't try to tense the muscles other than the ones intended, and it will make a huge difference in the result that you get from this.

When you do this, you might actually feel a different sensation when you relax, such as the blood flow to the arm, or even warmth of the feeling, and you may even start to realize as well that, when you're about to tense up, your warmth goes away. This is actually a great thing to learn since it allows you to become more mindful of how you respond to the different stimuli in life, and when you're about to get nervous or anxious about something.

At this point, do this for about 16 minutes or so, allowing you to relax each part of the body, one group of muscles at a time. Do this at least once a day, sometimes twice a day works wonders.

**Repetitive Statements**

This is something that can be used whether you're religious or not. Some people call this constant prayer, and it does have a religious focus, and a spirituality focus too, but that doesn't always have to be the case. It's good for those people who want to have something that is short, and effective to help with reducing stress, and anxiety.

What you do, is you practice focusing your breath, and you as a small phrase that comes from this. You focus on the phrase, and your mind immediately will think about this first and foremost, not worrying about anything else. It's a good one to try, and if you do have small phrases that help you, this is a great one to try for yourself.

**Applied Relaxation**

This is another type of relaxation developed by a Swedish physician, and it allows you to learn to relax quickly in certain circumstances, which allows for skills to develop based on each of the stages, and it usually takes a few stages to fully practice.

**What you do is follow the guide below:**

• Start with progressive muscle relaxation, learning to tense the muscle groups in a quicker manner, beginning with 18 minutes and you may notice it is being done in about 8-9 minutes.

• Release only relaxation. You tense and release the muscles a lot quicker

• Cue-controlled: it allows you to determine when you need to relax, and understanding the cues that are needed to relax the body

• Differential relaxation: allows you to learn how to relax during real-life situations, and how it allows you to isolate the muscles for each task

• Rapid relaxation: allows you to reduce your relaxation time over time to about 20-30 seconds which allows you to associate with the cues for relaxation, which allows the person to relax during normal, non-stressful situations

• Applied Relaxation: it uses the same techniques in before, but it also is used for stressful activities, including for those that have anxiety

Essentially, it's taking the progressive muscle relaxation and applying it to the moments when you know that you're suffering from anxiety. For example, if you know that something is going to make you anxious, you recognize the stimuli, and you work from there. It's quite miraculous how this can help you, and how you can, with this, understand the real reasoning behind why you react so that you can better handle that type of reaction, and learn to relax as well.

Learning relaxation techniques for anxiety is quite essential, and you'll realize over time that, once you master these, it's so much easier to manage, and you'll be much happier, and be able to reduce the stress that you feel by a lot as a result of this.

Breathing for Relaxation

Breathing for relaxation is a big part of guided meditation, and it's something that many people don't realize is a valuable skill for you to use in order to relax effectively. But, what's so special about breathing? How do you do it? Well, read on to find out.

Breathe!

You probably have been told when working to relax is to breathe or take a few breaths. This is often told when we're upset and worried. You might wonder why you should be told this when you're upset and worried, but it actually is beneficial when you're feeling anxious, and it can alter the speed of response to the body's breathing and anxiety. Diaphragmic is a breathing technique that is pretty helpful. It can create a developed feeling that actually communicates to our brain the element of safety.

I don't suggest using this immediately when you're super deep in an anxious moment, but, you should, if there is a tough situation, use this in order to make a smarter choice when trying to figure out what to do next.

Plus, breathing is actually helpful for calming down, and it's a vital part of relaxing the body when you're trying to de-stress. Being able to breathe after a long day can be really cathartic, and it's something that lots of times people don't even realize they forget to do.

Breathing with meditation is essential, and there are a few ways for you to breathe effectively in a meditative sense, and luckily, we'll tell you how to do it here.

**Diaphragmic Breathing**

Also known as Eupnea or belly breathing is a breathing technique that helps to strengthen your diaphragm. Learning to Breath from your diaphragm is useful as it helps to relax the body, the breathing, and the like. Lots of times, we actually don't breathe from our diaphragm, resulting in shorter breaths that don't bring oxygen-rich air to the body. This results in people taking breaths that don't help calm down the body, and they aren't refreshing. Luckily, you can learn to breathe from your diaphragm in this section, and we'll teach you how to here.

When you're using breathing for meditation using your diaphragm, you first and foremost want to sit with the feet planted on the floor or laying down. Put your hands right over your belly. From here, close your eyes, breathing in slowly and in a calm manner. Fill the belly with a normal breath, and don't breathe too heavily. You'll feel your hands move as you do breathe in like you're filling up a balloon. Don't lift the shoulders as you inhale, but instead, work on breathing into the stomach.

At this point, breathe out to the count of five. Slow the rate of exhaling. After you finish exhaling, you hold this for a couple of seconds before you breathe this in again. Continue to work to continue the pace and slowness of the breath that is here. Do this for about 10 or so minutes, and practice this twice daily for 10 minutes each time. Do this routine regularly to help with your own personal meditation.

You can couple this with focusing on the breathing, and when an intrusive thought comes in, you can actually eliminate that thought by acknowledging it, and of course, letting it stick around till it's gone but not obsessing over it. But, if that's too hard for you, do take some time to just focus on learning how to breathe in an effective manner. It's something that's essential for learning how to breathe via your diaphragm and is important.

Now, a couple of points to take away from it are as follows. You should focus on your breath speed rather than the depth of the breath. Don't catch your breath by taking in more profound ones, but instead, take it nice and slow.

Remember that with this, you won't be able just magically to turn off anxiety. That's not how this works, and instead, breathing will help you learn to relax and get through a tougher situation, and you can mostly use this as training to get into breathing in a calmer style with time.

Don't be afraid to practice this either. It takes a long time to master, but it does help immensely.

## 4-7-8 breathing

4-7-8 breathing technique is similar to breathing from your diaphragm but is kind of more of a timed step. It's good for people with anxiety and insomnia as it helps your mind and body to focus on your breath rather than thinking of your worries.

What you do to begin, is you can either sit or lay down, and keep your hand on your belly, and then keep the other on the chest, similar to how you breathe from your diaphragm. But, what you do, is when you breathe in slowly, are you take in slow, deep breaths that go straight to the belly, and from there, silently count to four whenever you breathe in.

At this point, instead of exhaling immediately, you then silently count from 1 to the number 7. When you hit 7, you breathe out completely, and you count from 1 all the way to 8, getting all of the air out of your lungs. Try to get all the air out by the time you reach eight. At this point, you then repeat this once again until you feel completely calm. With this one, I do suggest you journal how you feel at the end of this, and also how you feel. Chances are, you're going to feel much calmer than you did beforehand. This is great especially if you're in a situation where you need to focus on the numbers, and if you tend to be the type that needs that to be grounded, I suggest using this.

# Chapter 5    Meditation for Quieting Trauma, Depression, and Anxiety

After you have a physical wound on your body, there are four stages of healing that occur. These stages help to ensure that the wound doesn't get any worse and that it heals properly so that the rest of your body can still function. When we experience something traumatic or endure consistent depression and anxiety, it can be like a wound on your soul. These mental wounds don't have big ugly scars, like a scrape on your knee or cut on your face might. We have to remember, however, that these scars are still there.

These mental wounds are something that we still need to treat properly. In this meditation, we are going to help you understand how you can self-heal so that you can finally get the peace you need at night. Too often we lie awake thinking of the terrible things that we've experienced. How frequently do you find it almost impossible to actually get a restful night's sleep without waking up several times, playing a certain traumatic experience over and over again in your mind? You don't have to be a prisoner of your own experiences anymore. It is time to learn how you can best heal so that these wounds don't hurt.

Begin focusing on your breath right now. This is a great meditation to do before bed, but anytime that you need to be more relaxed, after dealing with trauma, anxiety, or depression is perfectly fine as well. Ensure that there are no distractions around you. You don't want any people, pets, music, sounds, sights, or anything else to keep you from being able to drift into a healthy and deep sleep. Feel as the air comes in and out of your body. Already, you can notice the way in which your body does what it can to ensure that you're getting taken care of properly. Even without us thinking about it, our bodies are constantly giving us the right things needed to survive.

We breathe, we digest, we live, we pump blood, and our heart beats. All of this continues to happen without us even having to think about it.

We do some of the work, but our body really comes in and does the rest. It knows exactly how to heal itself as well.

Think about this as you continue to breathe in and out. Breathe in through your nose and out through your mouth. This is a great way to keep you focused on your body. This is the method that you can use to ensure that you aren't thinking too hard about all that is negative for you.

Breathe in again, and out again. Breathe in through your nose for five, four, three, two, and one. Breathe out through your mouth for one, two, three, four, and five. Continue to breathe like this throughout the entire meditation.

When you get a cut or a scrape on your body, there are a few things that happen next in order to help you heal. The first step that happens after you cut yourself physically is that your body starts to go through hemostasis. This is the way that your body does what it can to stop the bleeding. At first, in this moment, your body is not concerned with healing. Your body is not going to immediately cover up that wound. All that matters is that the blood stops pouring out so that you don't have to lose any more of that.

This is incredibly powerful. This is what we do mentally. As soon as we experience something traumatic our bodies will try to stop it. It doesn't try to heal. It doesn't try to make sense of what's going on, and it doesn't try to give us a deep explanation to help further establish what we have been through. The only thing that our body does in this moment is try to make the trauma stop. It does whatever it can to make sure that we don't have to endure this pain anymore. Your body is incredibly powerful like this.

Understand what you might have gone through to make you try and stop the trauma. What experiences did you live through when your body did whatever it could to make this stop?

Did you try to self-sooth using outside sources? Maybe alcohol or drugs were able to stop the constant terror that ran through your mind.

Recognize this and remind yourself that whatever you have experienced is completely normal. This was your way your body tried to heal. We are past the stage now. Now it is time to move on to the next.

After you get a cut and the bleeding has stopped, what occurs next is inflammation. This inflammation is your body's way of fighting off any infection. It makes sure that the groundwork is in place for the actual restructuring of your skin to start.

Inflammation can be what occurs in us. This is when we are crying, when we are in pain, when we are screaming from anger, or when we are begging for things to stop. This is the stage that you might have gone through, but you are past this now. Your body was brave enough to pull you from this. You are so strong that you didn't have to deal with this anymore.

Your body did whatever it could to fight off this trauma and prevent it from happening again.

The point of this stage is to start a new growth process. You have moved past the initial fear and shock of what happened, and instead, you're looking for a way to heal. Unfortunately, not all of us understand the way that we are able to heal ourselves. This is when some things can get a little trickier. You are working through this now. You are fighting off this infection from ever coming back and taking over.

Next is proliferation. This is when the wound can start to close. Finally, it is not a sore spot anymore. This is the part that we need to focus on. You are focused on moving forward now. You understand that this wound is closing. It is finally healing. The skin is connected to itself once again to make sure that nothing can get in and nothing can get out.

Finally, in the stage of healing, your wound can form something new. This is when there might be a scar.

This is when you could be experiencing a reshaping of a physical part of your body. This is what happens to our soul. After we've experienced something traumatic, we never go back to the exact same way that things used to be. Instead, we only move forward and move on to something greater and better in the end.

Some people's wounds might heal incorrectly. They might let it become scar tissue on their soul, stopping another thing from functioning properly. You are not going to let this happen. You are healing now. You are feeling that wound finally close up. You don't have to let the feelings and emotions that you had at the time pour out anymore.

You're not closing things up so that you never deal with it again. You are simply closing it up because you are stronger and better now. You are moving past these challenging emotions. No longer do you have the challenging thoughts and feelings that used to pop up so frequently in the past.

The thing about scar tissue is that it will never be the same. Some scars will heal perfectly normally, and we don't even have to think about it. Then, there are plenty of other scars that can leave huge marks that can't be looked past. Eventually you'll get used to it. It is a part of you now, and this does not have to be so ugly. We don't have to consider scars as something scary or grotesque. They are simply another marking on our body. How many marks do you have simply from not even realizing that they are there?

Maybe there's a freckle on your cheek or a little cut on your arm from when you were a child and fell off your bike. Maybe you have some acne from when you were a teenager, struggling with the constant constellation of pimples across your face. Perhaps you can't grow hair on a certain patch on your body because of the scar. Maybe there's a big ugly lump on your leg that you hate to look at.

Whatever these are, we don't have to be afraid of them just like you don't have to fear the scar that is on your soul. You are moving on and past this now into a happier and healthier place. This scar is part of what makes you beautiful. Think of all the markings on a physical object that you see. Maybe you pull a little penny out of your change purse and notice all the small markings on this.

You can see all the scrapes and scratches along the face of the penny.

Each of these indicates something that it has gone through. It is a story; it is something that it came from. It is part of who it is. There is no going back or trying to erase it. This isn't going to help the wound heal. You have to let it heal properly to make it more manageable to handle later on.

Imagine just trying to cover up that wound. Imagine just putting makeup or a big Band-Aid over something that was infected. This is only going to make it worse. This isn't going to help you heal. Instead, the wound festers and it gets bigger and bigger.

Think about picking a scab and not being able to let it heal. This doesn't do it any good. It just makes it bigger and bigger and makes the scar deeper and deeper.

Let yourself heal naturally. You deserve to feel okay. What happened to you is not your fault. You don't have to hold on to these thoughts. We often remind ourselves of what we went through and this can make it hard to feel better. Make yourself feel good. Let yourself be happy. It's okay to experience good emotions even after constant years of feeling something so negative. Of course, it's not easy. Of course, this is not going to be a simple task.

This is something challenging. It is going to be a daily process that you have to work through, but it is going to be so worth it in the end. One day you will be able to look back on all of your struggles and your trauma and recognize that it has made you the person that you are today. You can grow and prosper from it. It does not have to be like a chain that keeps you strapped to the ground. You can spread your wings and be free. Feel yourself breathing in and out once again.

Breathe in good feelings and happiness. Breathe out the toxic negativity that has stuck around with you for so long. Remind yourself that with each breath you take, you are reminded at how alive and how strong and how brave you really are.

Each time you let air pass through your body, you are doing something good for it. You are taking care of yourself. You are loved. It doesn't matter who else loves you in this moment because you are loved by yourself and that is what is most important in the end.

You were brave and free. You are not tied just to the traumatic things that have happened to you. These are important because they can make up who you are. They give you a new perspective, and you have ideas that other people will never be able to experience. You understand evil and suffering on a different level.

You know what it feels like to hurt so much.

You recognize true pain, and not everyone will be able to say that. Of course, you might wish that you could be free from these experiences.

Perhaps you think about all the ways that you could become somebody who doesn't have to deal with challenging emotions. Maybe you envy those with easy carefree lives. Of course, that might be better, but we can never know. We will never understand because of our scars, and that is not a bad thing. These scars make us beautiful. They make us who we are. We can learn and grow and heal from them. They can teach us things. They remind us of what we've been through.

We recognize now that we are such an amazing person. These scars remind us of how resilient we are. They give us the recognition that we are able to take something so painful and grow from it. This scar does not destroy us. It is not the opening or the beginning of the end. It is the start of something new. It is a reminder that we will be better in the end because of this.

We know what true struggle is, and that means we recognize what real reward is. We have an appreciation for things like no other. We can have gratitude for the good because we have experienced so much bad.

Remind yourself of this. Recognize these emotions and let yourself relax. Let yourself be happy, free, calm, and collected. This is how you are going to heal. This is healthy for you. This is what you need.

Breathe in again and breathe out. Breathe in and breathe out. Feel the air travel so gently through your body. Let yourself heal and be happy.

As we count down from 20, remember to focus on your breathing.

20, 19, 18, 17, 16, 15, 14, 13, 12, 11, 10, 9, 8, 7, 6, 5, 4, 3, 2 and 1

It is okay to still hurt. It is okay to feel pain.

But you also need to relax.

We are now going to move on to a part where you can completely relax. When we reach one, you will have no thoughts passing through your mind.

We are going to help you drift deep into sleep now so that your traumas and triggers don't keep you up all night.

There is nothing but darkness around you. Now this does not make you scared, it simply reminds you of the significant life that you have.

You are a human being on this earth, and you are here as yourself. You are an individual, and you're strong. No matter what comes your way, you are going to be able to work through it. You have to get to sleep now so that you can perform as best as you can with all that you do.

It is okay to let yourself be relaxed. You do not have to be afraid anymore. Nothing is going to hurt you. No one is going to harm you. Nothing is going to scare you. You will not be haunted all night by the things that give you so much terror.

Count down now again. Let yourself get deeper and deeper into sleep.

10, 9, 8, 7, 6, 5, 4, 3, 2, and 1.

….. and you're closer and closer to sleep now.

Count again.

10, 9, 8, 7, 6, 5, 4, 3, 2, 1 and you're closer and closer and closer to sleep.

One more time we are going to count down from twenty.

As we reach one, you will either drift off into sleep or move on to another meditation. You are safe, you are protected, you are healthy, and you are peaceful.

What happened to you in the past plays no role in this sleep now. All that matters is the moment. This moment is one where you can be completely relaxed.

You are not in any harm's way. You are at peace.

20, 19, 18, 17, 16, 15, 14, 13, 12, 11, 10, 9, 8, 7, 6, 5, 4, 3, 2 and 1

# Chapter 6     30 Minute Guided Meditation for Sleep, Relaxation, & Stress Relief

**[Introduction- Stretch and positioning: 3 minutes]**

Before we begin, I'd like you to take a couple of minutes to prepare yourself for a restful sleep.

Prepare your room by turning off any devices that might be a distraction. You may need to put your phone in another room if you are tempted to check it repeatedly. Turn off the TV or any music that is playing. You want to set the stage for a night of rest and relaxation. Dim the lights.

Lie down, on your back and settle into a position that is comfortable for you. If you are not comfortable lying on your back, you might want to put a rolled blanket under your knees. Make sure that your head and neck are supported as well.

If it is comfortable for you, try moving your head back and forth and turning it side to side to loosen up your neck muscles.

Let it relax back into a comfortable position

Wiggle your shoulders and let them fall back into a relaxed position

Keeping your buttocks on the bed, move your hips a bit and then let them fall back into a relaxed position.

You want your body to be in a neutral and comfortable position so:

Make sure that your chin is not pointing too far up. Tuck in in just a bit to allow the neck to lengthen and the jaw to relax.

Tuck your shoulders underneath you and then let them relax into a natural position

Let your hands rest at your sides, palms up or down, or on your abdomen.

Let your legs relax, your feet and knees may roll out when they are relaxed. Try not to hold them in any specific position, just let them fall naturally.

*Pause to allow participants a couple minutes to adopt a comfortable position.*

**[Intention setting and focus on breathing: 10 minutes]**

You may find that you will doze during this meditation. That is ok. Don't force yourself to stay awake if you feel that you are sleepy.

Close your eyes lightly. For this time, you aren't going to try to do anything. There is no need to worry about things that happened today or things that might happen tomorrow. Right now, all you need to do is to be here, in your body, on your bed letting your mind do what it needs to do to relax for a good night's sleep.

Thank yourself for taking this time for self-care. You deserve a night of restful sleep and to wake up feeling refreshed and ready for the day. This is one thing that you can do that is just for yourself. No guilt, no worries.

Know that whatever worries you and stops you from sleeping won't be fixed by keeping you awake.

Know that no matter how you slept last night, or the night before, you can sleep well tonight. This is the only night that matters.

During this meditation, each time you find your mind drifting, notice where it's gone and gently tell yourself to come back to being right here, right now. There is no need to judge what your mind is thinking about or that you have become distracted. This is what our brains are designed to do and most of us spend all day trying to think about many things all at once. It is not easy to undo years of training and it probably won't be undone today but you've already started doing the best thing that you can do to unclutter your mind.

Breath in and out naturally a few times.

Think about your breath but try not to change it. This is your natural breath. You do this all day without thinking about it. For just a few minutes, focus on this activity. So easy it happens without any thought or effort.

*Pause a minute for reflection*

Take a few deep breaths and exhale whatever tension you feel. Inhale slowly and really feel where the air is going. It is normal to breath less than we can. Right in this moment, you want to breath as fully as possible.

Take a deep breath and feel the air as it flows through your nostrils, down into your lungs and fully into your abdomen. Breathe in as deeply as you can.

Exhale slowly, pushing the air out, first from your abdomen and then from your lungs.

Think about any areas of tightness you may have had when you took that breath. If it felt stuck anywhere, feel what it would be like to relax that area.

You are going to take a few deep breaths again and think about relaxing into the breath. I will be giving you instructions for relaxation but don't feel that you need to match the pace of your breath with my instructions. Just keep breathing deeply and try to apply the instructions with each breath.

When you exhale, don't push out the air so much that you are pulling in your stomach. Let the exhale come to a natural end with your body feeling relaxed and empty of air.

On your next deep inhale, feel the flow through your nostrils, down behind your jaw into your throat. Sometimes people tighten their throat when breathing deeply. Try to tuck your chin, just a bit, to lengthen your neck relax your jaw and think about opening your throat to allow the air to pass freely through and into your lungs.

Exhale slowly, feeling the air flow out of your body.

*Pause a minute for reflection*

Inhale deeply again, feeling the air through your nostrils and throat and into your lungs. Relax your chest and let your lungs expand with the breath. Think about opening your lungs out and not up. If you feel your shoulders rising, think about relaxing them back down and to the sides while letting your lungs push out with air.

Exhale fully and try that again. Inhale deeply into your lungs, relaxing your shoulder down and away from your ears and letting your lungs fill until they are large and full.

Exhale naturally.

*Pause a minute for reflection*

On your next deep inhale, feel the airflow from your nostril, down your throat and into your lungs. Feel your abdomen rise as you fill your lungs. Relax your stomach and let it push out. Don't worry, no one is watching. Use your stomach to help your lungs fill more fully. A lot of us aren't used to relaxing our stomachs this way. We don't like to push it out and look fat but know that no one is watching you right now.

Exhale naturally, relax your stomach and try that again. Inhale deeply, feeling the air in your lungs and your abdomen pushing out. Relaxing your shoulders and letting your stomach push out.

Take three more deep breaths at your own pace, feel for any remaining areas of tension. Meet those areas without judgment and try to relax them. Don't worry if they still feel tight. Just take note of them as you move your attention elsewhere.

Let you breath relax and become natural again.

*Pause a minute for reflection*

**[Bodyscan: 10 minutes]**

As your body relaxes, it may begin to feel heavy. Feel how it rests on the bed. You are supported in this meditation by the things around you. They hold you and allow you to do the work you need to do to unclutter your mind.

Like your breath, your body may hold areas of tension that distract you. As we scan the body, we will try to release these areas and achieve a fuller relaxation. When you notice tension, try to relax those muscles. You may find that a small stretch and release of the muscles helps reduce the tension. This doesn't have to be a big movement. It is something that resets the muscle memory into one of relaxation rather than tension.

Bring your attention to the top of your head. Focus on what that feels like. Maybe it's warm or maybe you feel a breeze. If you don't think about it much, it might be hard to feel the top of your head. Imagine it touching the air around you. You might feel something strongly, like heat or a breeze. Whatever you feel, or don't feel, is ok. Just notice whatever it is, without judgment.

*Pause a minute for reflection*

Move your attention to your cheeks and around your mouth. Notice if you are holding tension in either of these places. Think about what to would feel like to let that tension go. Try bringing your lips into a soft small smile. This smile is mostly internal. It always feels better to smile and helps to relax your whole face. Don't worry if this all feels a little funny, just relax and let it happen or not without judgment.

*Pause a minute for reflection*

Now bring your attention to your neck and shoulders. These are very common areas for storing stress and tension. If you keep them tight, you may not even be able to imagine what they would feel like relaxed. Try shrugging your shoulders and tucking them back. Move your head back and forth a little bit. If any of these actions hurts, stop. Let your shoulders feel heavy and fall away from your neck. Notice whatever you feel in your neck and shoulders without judgment. However much you relax them is more than they were relaxed before!

*Pause a minute for reflection*

Focus on your heart area, stomach, and abdomen. Notice if you are holding any tension on those areas. Nerves and worries like to settle there. You can let those go for now. If you need them, they will come back but, for this small amount of time, you can just let them go. Thinking about your worries may have reminded you about something you need to start or finish (or start and finish). You have already promised yourself that you will get to those things when you are finished with this. You can let the wait for just a few more minutes while you prepare your mind for them. Holding tension in your stomach won't help them to get done. Try to imagine your chest and stomach relaxed and not distracting you from things you want to focus on.

*Pause a minute for reflection*

Move your attention to your arms. They might feel heavy to you that is how they are when they are relaxed. Let them rest however is comfortable to you. Notice if you have any tension in your hands and stretch your fingers just a bit to let that go. Let them relax again, resting on your legs or the floor.

*Pause a minute for reflection*

Bring your attention into your lower back and pelvis. You've been sitting still for a few minutes and may find that you are tight. Feel free to wiggle a bit to get comfortable and release any tension that may be in your lower back. Notice any areas of tension in your pelvis. Let any tension go without letting yourself slump or slouch.

*Pause a minute for reflection*

Now move your attention to your legs and feet. Sometimes, we are so used to holding ourselves up with our legs that we don't even notice the tension we have in our thighs. Lt the fall naturally while keeping your feet connected to the floor. If you are lying down, let your knees and feet fall naturally to the side. You may want to stretch or wiggle them a bit to feel the relaxation.

Take three deep breaths at your own pace, linger a bit on the exhale but don't force it.

Feel what this state of full relaxation feels like. Maybe you haven't felt this relaxed in a while. Know that you can create this for yourself at any time.

*Pause for moment for reflection*

**[Conclusion: 7 minutes]**

Shift your focus back to your breath. Let your breathing become natural and notice the inhale and exhale. Try not to force it. If you find yourself breathing slower or faster than normal, notice that and try to let the need to control the breath go. Normally, you don't think much about your breathing so it's common for people to change how they breathe when they start to pay attention to it.

This is a light focus on your breath.

It's just in …. And out…..

One breath, in….. And out

When your mind drifts, notice that you have become distracted and, without judging, bring your attention back to this one breath.

Focus on just this breath…..

Take each breath one at a time.

As you end this meditation, thank yourself for taking this time to prepare yourself and settle your mind and body for a restful night's sleep. It might not feel like it, but you have taken an important step towards clearing your mind and practicing relaxation. This will help you to let go of whatever thoughts or worries might prevent you for sleeping well.

Know that you can achieve this level of relaxation every night before bed. When you want this, just take a moment to feel your breath and remind yourself that worries and tension are just distractions that you can put aside while you focus on more important things. Whenever you feel them creeping into your mind, bring your attention back to the breath.

Inhale

Exhale

Take one more deep breath and feel the weight of your body on the bed. This is rest. This is how you replenish.

Let yourself feel this fully and completely

Let yourself rest.

# Chapter 7    Deep Sleep Techniques

## Meditation to Overcome Insomnia

Whether you find it difficult to sleep at night as a result of stress, tiredness, work or several other factors, or you find your sleep unsatisfactory, you might be suffering from insomnia. Insomnia is commonly called difficulty falling asleep, or staying awake, and there two types of insomnia.

Acute insomnia is mostly caused as a result of lifestyle, or circumstances. A security officer on night duty will find it difficult to fall asleep on duty, likewise a first-time dad may find it difficult to fall asleep thinking of his precious wife in labor.

While, chronic insomnia is a complicated type of insomnia. There is no known underlying cause, yet the individual finds it difficult to either fall asleep, or sleep at night for long hours. Such person may also experience disrupted sleep, for more than 3 times a week.

Experiencing insomnia regularly causes mood disturbances, fatigue, stress and difficulty concentrating. Although, insomnia can be caused by factors like anxiety, work related stress, lifestyle, and sicknesses. However, the approach to overcome insomnia is not easy for some persons, yet there is one possible way to overcome not just insomnia but enjoy a long, satisfactory sleep for the rest of your life.

## How Does Meditation Cure Insomnia

Meditation is a relaxation technique worth trying, which can help improve your sleep, make you fall asleep easily and also make your sleep satisfactory, such that you wake up feeling refreshed. Meditation harmonizes the mind and body, and also influences the brain and the way it functions. The effect of meditation on your mind and body is that you become calm, and relaxed afterwards.

## Effect of Meditation on Insomnia

During meditation, the mind is focused on one thing, which prevents the mind from wandering. Your mind and thoughts are brought to the now moment during meditation. Hence, anxiety disappears and it becomes easier to fall asleep.

During the meditation, your mind and body are been connected to each other, and they both become relaxed and calm, which helps you sleep as soon as you get in bed.

Furthermore, meditation helps boost the hormone called melatonin that regulates the sleep and wake cycle. Without stress, the melatonin level is usually at its peak at night to ensure you get a sound, and restful sleep. However, the presence of stress among other factors that causes insomnia, the melatonin level drastically reduces, thereby insomnia occurs. With meditation, the melatonin level increases because stress has been reduced, and the body is in a relaxed state.

**Meditation Techniques for Insomnia**

If you want to experience an undisrupted sleep, an intense meditation must be done frequently. There are different techniques of meditating for insomnia and understanding process help us to get started immediately.

•     Cognitive shuffling

Cognitive shuffling is a simple meditation technique that can be done alone. It is simply a do-it-yourself technique that shuffles your thoughts to sleep. Here is how cognitive shuffling works, when you lie on your bed, your mind is likely to be filled with different thoughts from your daily activities. You can be worried, and anxious about your bills, relationship, the next day activities, such that you find it difficult to fall asleep. The effect of this shuffling on the brain is it tricks the mind to get into a dreaming state.

Tips to Practice Cognitive Shuffling

- Firstly, getting in bed is important

- Right there on your bed, avoid focusing your concerns. Let your deadline be, the bills, the complicated issue at work. Let it all be.

- Now that your mind is free from your fears and worries, create a new engagement like imagining objects, places, names or movies to meditate on. You can imagine different things, like a teddy bear, a fish, a dog, the sky, the rainbow, or the ocean. Note that, the items you are imagining should not be threatening or scary. For instance, instead of imagining an ocean because you have the fear of water, you can imagine the rainbow or the sky with beautiful stars.

- Ensure your eyes are closed before you begin the cognitive shuffling process.

- Process should be repeated if you are still awake, until you run out of words.

•     Sa Ta Na Ma (Mantra)

Sa Ta Na Ma is a powerful meditation technique that works on the brain and its functions to reduce risk of depression and other mental illness. It is a mantra that is usually recited in 3 voices; the singing voice which stands for the action voice.

The whispered voice which stands for your inner voice, and

The silent voice is known as your spirit's voice.

SA TA NA MA chant describes the evolutionary aspect of the universe. Each word in the chant has a meaning.

SA means the beginning.

TA means existence and creativeness

NA means death or the end of life

MA means rebirth

The effect of this mantra is displayed by a balance in emotions, and a settled mind.

Practical steps to Sa Ta Na Ma

- Find a comfortable position. You can sit down or lie down.

- Decide on how many minutes you want to recite the mantra.

- Breathe in and out through your nose and mouth and ensure you sigh after this breathing exercise is heard.

- Close your eyes properly, and place your hands either on your lap, or knee. Make sure your palm is facing up.

- Begin chanting slowly, and press the thumb of your hands, with your four fingers. Count your fingers each starting from the thumb to recite the mantra.

- Keep reciting the chant as a calm and slow pace

During recitation, you have to follow the principles of the mantra.

When you mention SA, you count from your index to your thumb

You count from your middle finger to your thumb when you sing TA

You count from your ring finder to thumb when you recite NA

And final you should count from your pinky finger to the thumb when you mention MA.

- Still in that position, sing SA TA NA MA in a loud voice, your voice should be audible, and ensure you move each of your fingers with each sound. The more you sing, the more you feel relaxed and energetic. However, your soul and spirit should feel relaxed and enjoy the sensation which is moving through your body and mind.

- When you feel relaxed, shift your focus and start singing in a whisper voice. At this point, energy is flowing through the body, waist, and knee.

- Next, be focused on silence. Continue counting your fingers and silently repeat the mantra to yourself.

- After singing the mantra completely, breathe in and breathe out with your arms wide open, and lift the hand above your head. Release your hands down, and exhale again. Repeat process until you feel refreshed or drowsy.

**What to Expect When Meditating To Fall Asleep**

Your expectations when meditating to fall asleep is most likely to have a sound and deep sleep at night, except you are uncertain about the benefits of meditation. Meditation for sleep is similar to other kind of meditation; however, the approach to each of these meditations is what matters.

When meditating, your meditation technique determines what you will have to do. Albeit, you can start preparing for your meditation exercise, by breathing in and out, lying flat on your back. If you are having a guided meditation, all you need to do is follow the instructions instead of been worried about what to do and what not to do.

Furthermore, all you should when meditating to fall asleep is sleep, but try to avoid any form of distractions.

How to Meditate Before Sleep

There are two ways you can meditate before going to bed, it can be a mindful meditation where you pay more attention to your body and mind, and also having a guided meditation where someone leads you through the process of meditation.

Mindfulness meditation can be done alone, in your own room house and house. While guided meditation is a very easy meditation, it is just for you to follow and listen to instructions from a guide.

## Guided Meditation Tips for Insomnia

Guided meditation is the form of meditation you engage in with the help of a tutor, or instructor. Ensure that you will not be disturbed, during the course of this meditation.

- Lay down on your back, preferably on your bed or mat. Make sure you are comfortable on whatever you are lying on.

- Close your eyes and prepare your mind for the meditation you are about to engage in.

- Breathe in and out, ensure that your breathing out is audible such that it looks like you breathing out heavily. Make your body feel the heaviness, after which your body will be relaxed.

- Pay more attention to your breathing, and you feel easiness. A natural breathing process.

- At this point, you will feel your body is relaxed. Feel the way your breath travels through your lungs, and hold your breath. As this is happening, you will begin to feel relaxation in your body.

- You can begin to breathe normally right now, and as you breathe you feel your muscles, joints, and back relaxed.

- Pay more attention to your stomach area right now, where your abdominal muscles are present. Tighten the muscles in your abdomen, and hold your breath for 10 seconds and release your muscles. During this release, feel the difference the tightness of your abdominal muscle and the relaxation of these muscles.

- Repeat the above process 5 times.

- Breathe in and out, tighten your abdomen and release it to relaxation.

Feet

- Divert your attention to your feet, and make them relaxed. The relaxation should be from your toes to your ankles. Tighten your toes and feet, and feel them become heavy and relaxed.

- Focus on your nails, feel them relaxed and let go.

- Pay attention to your thigh area, and feel them relaxed.

- Again, focus on your waist, lower and upper back, joints and feel them relaxed. You will feel the feel heavy, and very relaxed

Upper limbs

- At this point, focus your attention on your arms. Feel them heavy and relaxed.

- Get a sense of how heavy your arm is, and feel the relaxation shift to your elbow, wrist, and fingers become very relaxed.

Face, neck and facial muscles

- Shift your focus to your facial muscles, neck and face.

-       Every muscle in your face, your cheeks and chin becomes relaxed, and your entire body is now relaxed.

A deeper meditation for the abdomen

-       Locate your center, which is your abdominal region. Imagine there is a bowl on your abdomen. Slowly see the bowl rolling over your abdomen area, and it relaxes every muscle the bowl rolls in contact with.

-       The bowl now moves slowly from your abdomen area to your right hip carefully and softly massaging the muscles of the hips it comes in contact to.

-       Massaging back and forth all the muscles in your abdomen.

-       The ball continues to roll over to your knee, and around your knee. You can feel the tension on your navel melting away. Roll the ball slowly to your toe, and over to your toes, from your small toes to the big toes.

Every part of your body this ball comes in contact with feel the part of your body relaxing.

-       Now feel the ball begins to roll upwards away from your toes again. Massaging and reducing tension around your toes, knees, ankles and rolls over to your center, your abdominal area.

-       Again, this balls rolls to your left thigh, and your knee, massaging both the back and front of your knee.

With your ball you move this ball to wherever you choose, and how long you want it to be.

-       With this ball, massage your knee, and ankle and toes. This ball touches every muscle in your toes, it gently massages them and at this point, you feel your muscle relax.

-       Feel the ball roll back up your leg, your knee and thigh muscle and arriving back at your center.

-       Shift the focus of the ball to the base of your spinal cord. Allow the ball rest there for 5 seconds, and allow it move up your spine, and near your heart. At this point, you can feel the ball massaging the internal organs in your body. The ball massages the heart, and you feel relaxed.

-       The ball rolls to your throat area, and the back of your neck area. You feel your neck area relaxing after the ball massages it. You feel tension reducing around your neck area.

-       The ball travels down your arm, and to your wrist. The ball gently massages your wrist, and fingers.

- You feel the ball roll up your arm, to your shoulder and neck. It travels down to your elbow, forearm, and wrist and into the palm of your hands.

- Allow the ball gently massage your palm, and fingers. The ball moves up your arm, shoulder and face and as it reaches up in your face, the ball splits into a hundred tiny balls. You feel them travel around your face, to your eyes, eyebrow, cheeks, chin, teeth, tongue and teeth.

- You feel the ball massaging your face and every part of your face. At this point, you should enjoy this facial massage.

- I want you to imagine as you are lying down the ceiling of your house. Your eyes is still closed, so imagine the ceiling of your room opening itself up, and the roof also opens itself open.

- Still looking at this opening, you will see the beautiful white sky. The sky is clear, bright, and the moon is out and also full, filled with stars. This is a magical peaceful night. You are alone, safe in the beautiful part of your house.

- Watch the twinkling and beautiful little stars, looking down on you and you are enjoying the peace of the night.

- You look again at the stars again, the little ones that are thousands of miles away are not shining so beautiful like the big star closer to you, that is looking at you directly from the sky.

- You are looking deep into galaxy, beyond time, you see a million other stars waiting for you and shining at you.

- Take a deep breath. Breathe in a rich air from the infinite and beautiful galaxy filled with stars.

- Feel yourself been a part of these stars, there is no separation between you and them. Feel you are already a part of this wonderful galaxy.

- As you experience this, you become a shooting star, shining across the galaxy like others.

- Slowly you begin to fade into the sky, into the unending space and galaxy.

- You are living in the wonders of this space, where there is neither time, past or future. You feel you are the stars, the moon, and you occupy the pace between the planets.

- You are floating off slowly, as you travel across this universe; you feel your body wants to drift away. You feel peace, wholeness, and love.

- When you are ready, and feel relaxed, you can let go of the galaxy. When you drift off, you will drift into a peaceful and wonderful sleep.

# Chapter 8    Empty Mind Meditation

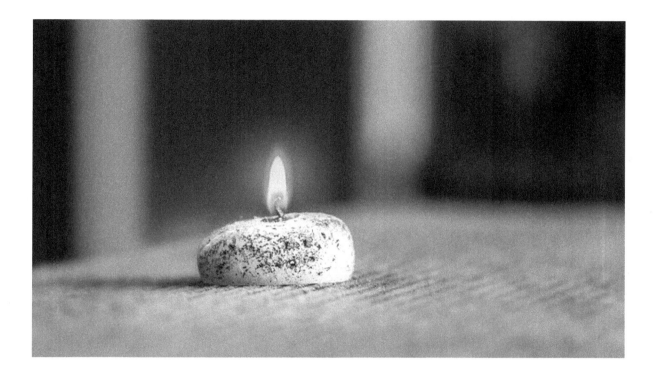

Empty Mind Meditation is one of the more challenging forms of meditation as it requires you to still your mind to the point that you are thinking about nothing. To many people this may seem, at first hearing about it, to be impossible, but with much practice it is entirely possible for anyone to master Empty Mind Meditation.

First, it is recommended that you begin with one of the easier forms of meditation, such as Breathing Meditation or Mantra Meditation, until you are completely comfortable with the basic principles and techniques of meditation. Focusing on one thing and only one thing is hard enough for most people -- focusing on nothing can be even harder.

The key to Empty Mind Meditation is the ability to train your mind to be aware of when you have a thought and then banish the thought from your mind. It is best to practice Breathing Meditation, Mantra Meditation, and Mindfulness Meditation before attempting Empty Mind Meditation if you are looking for quick results as you will already be familiar with techniques employed to aid you in focusing on one thing and nothing else. With Empty Mind Meditation, that one thing is nothing.

It is recommended that you begin Empty Mind Meditation by focusing on your breath, much like Breathing Meditation. Unlike Breathing Meditation, however, eventually you will stop paying attention to everything, including your breath. You may attempt Empty Mind Meditation in any Asana of your choosing so long as it will not distract you from thinking of nothing (i.e. your feel falling asleep, general discomfort, etc.). Start a session of Breathing Meditation, and once you have been able to still your thoughts to a suitable point and are focused solely on your breath, stop keeping track of the number of seconds that you are breathing in and out as well as the number of times that you have inhaled and exhaled. You will notice that at first your mind wanders, and this is to be expected. Empty Mind Meditation takes practice, and one of the best methods of attaining results is to keep track of the number of times that your mind wanders.

At first you may not even be aware that your mind has wandered, thinking about something for several seconds before realizing that you have thought of something. When this happens, it is best to finish the thought as to allow it to pass from your mind. When you have done this, resume your Breathing Meditation and, when you are comfortable, again stop focusing on your breath. It may take some time before you are able to focus on nothing at all for a sustained period of time, and that is why it is important to keep some sort of a record of the number of times you notice your mind wandering during each session. If you are practicing Empty Mind Meditation properly you will notice that the number will slowly decrease. Eventually you should have a session without a single break.

It is important to keep in mind that there is no right or wrong way to perform Empty Mind Meditation so long as you focus on nothing. What is meant by this is that is perfectly acceptable to begin your session as Breathing Meditation or Mantra Meditation and work your way towards Empty Mind Meditation as long as you are able to get to a point where you are able to focus on nothing.

If you have even entered a trance state during any of your meditative practices, you will have experienced Empty Mind Meditation. In this state you will be unaware of any physical sensations, completely forgetting about your body, your thoughts, and time. You will seem to exist as a pure consciousness. This is known in the Sanskrit as Samadhi. The origin and definition of the word Samadhi is a topic of debate, but it is clear that Samadhi is a trance state where the one meditating has reached one-pointedness and a perfect stillness of mind.

Most people may not realize it, but we sometimes find ourselves in a state of Empty Mind Meditation without being aware of it. Have you ever found yourself 'spacing out', as it is referred to? That is, completely unaware of anything going on around you. You may seem to an outside observer to be in a state of deep thought, but in truth were someone to ask you what you were thinking about you would tell them that you didn't know, or perhaps nothing. While the reason or reasons behind this remain somewhat unclear (the effects of certain drugs have been known to have this effect, as have certain illnesses, but a reason for it to occur spontaneously and naturally has yet to be agreed upon), what is clear is that it is entirely possible for one to enter a trance state without ever even having attempted to attain one.

The key to mastering meditation in any or all of its varied forms is the same as the key to mastering anything -- time and practice. If you expect to sit down and immediately enter into a trance state, you are going to be disappointed when it doesn't happen. If you think five minutes of meditation are going to enlighten you or make you feel better (physically, mentally, or spiritually) I have some bad news for you, because it won't.

If, however, you are willing to put in the time and the effort required to gain the benefits of any type of meditation, I can guarantee that you will notice improvement not only in your ability to meditate but also with your memory, awareness, self-control, brain function, how well you sleep, and much, much more. There are a nearly limitless number of benefits to setting aside a little time every day to meditate. You should always try to meditate at the same time so that your body and mind associate that time with meditation. This will actually make it easier for you to enter a trance state faster because you will already be prepared to do so. Make sure to keep notes of all your sessions that include your Asana, Mantra (if one was used), length of the session, and the number of breaks in focus. This way you will be able to see if a particular pose or a specific word seem to be helping you to make progress or hindering you from doing so.

Lastly, if you're having trouble with any form of meditation, don't get discouraged. Keep practicing, and in time you will be a master of not only the practice of meditation but of yourself as well.

# Chapter 9    Mindful Meditation

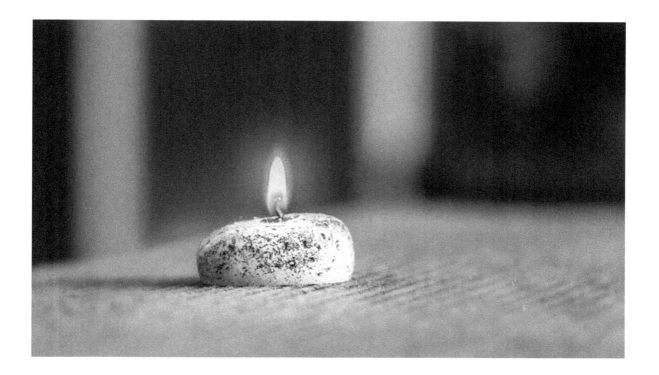

Mindfulness Meditation refers to any meditation in which you focus on the present moment and everything that goes along with it. Instead of focusing on a single thing, as is the case with most forms of meditation, Mindfulness Meditation requires you to focus on everything both within and without you at any given moment. Every sound, smell, taste, touch, and (if you choose to meditate with your eyes open) sight should be focused on and analyzed so that you may become aware of its true meaning and become one with its essence. The same goes for every natural function of the body as well.

The goal of Mindfulness Meditation is to become more aware of not only the world around you but also your inner self, giving you a better understanding of the way the world works as well as a fuller knowledge of your inner self and who you really are. This is also the form of meditation most often associated with improved memory, bodily health, and general awareness. Mindfulness Meditation is often practiced in a seated position, and there are many Asanas -- or body postures -- that are perfect for a session of Mindfulness Meditation.

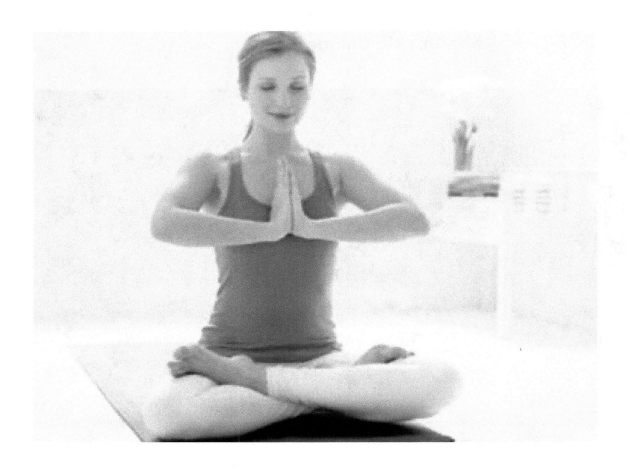

The most well-known seated Asana is Padmasana but is also known as the Lotus. To get into this position, begin by sitting on the ground with your legs crossed (commonly referred to as Indian Style). Take one foot and place it on top of the opposite thigh with the bottom of the foot facing upward, then take the opposite foot and place it on top of the other thigh, again with the bottom of the foot facing upward. Your knees should be touching the ground and, as with most any Asana, your spine should be straight.

This pose may be difficult for some people to get into, especially those carrying a little extra weight. If you are having difficulty getting into the Lotus, you may always try the Half Lotus. The Half Lotus is exactly the same as the Lotus except you only place one foot on top of the opposite thigh instead of both of them. The other foot remains in the position it was in when you originally sat down and crossed your legs.

Another good pose for Mindfulness Meditation is the Dragon. To get into the Dragon pose, sit on your knees with your feet under your buttocks. Your buttocks should be resting on your heels and your toes should be pointed in the same direction, either out away from the body or in toward the body. Make sure that your big toes are touching and that you keep your spine straight. Your hands should be resting on your knees to help support your weight and keep your body propped up and your head should be facing forward.

There is a downside to most seated Asanas, and that is that eventually your feet begin to go numb. This is to be expected, and though at first it may be distracting you should be able to learn to ignore it without it affecting your session. In fact, in the case of Mindfulness Meditation, the sensation of your feet going numb could be used as your focus, so it is not necessarily a bad thing; but if you were practicing Breathing Meditation or Mantra Meditation it may make it very difficult for you to concentrate.

Some of the most popular forms of Mindfulness Meditation involve meditating on the Tattva (the Sanskrit for 'Truth') or the Chakra ('Wheel'). According to tradition there are five Tattva. These are Akasa, or Spirit; Vayu, or Air; Tejas, or Fire; Apas, or Water; and Prithvi, or Earth.

Each of the Tattva are represented by a specific shape and color, and to meditate on them you must be aware of both of those things. Akasa is represented as a black egg, Vayu is represented as a blue circle, Tejas is represented as a red triangle, Apas is represented as a silver crescent, and Prithvi is represented as a yellow square.

To meditate upon one of them, simple choose the one you wish to focus on. However, unlike other forms of meditation where you try not to focus on anything but the chosen object, in Mindfulness Meditation you are attempting to go beyond the basic form of something in order to gain the understanding of its true meaning. With the Tattva it is important that you focus only on the color and shape chosen to the exclusion of all other mental forms and images, but it is also important that you realize that you are not focusing on the colors or shapes themselves but what these colors and shapes truly mean. It is a somewhat abstract concept, but with time and practice you will develop a better knowledge of what exactly it means to go beyond merely imagining an object.

If, however, you wish to meditate on something more directly related to inner knowledge of self, the Chakra points are probably your best starting point. In Hindu beliefs, the Chakra is what is known as a 'subtle body', sometimes referred to as a 'body of light' in other schools of thought.

It should be remembered that, while the Chakra points correspond to various places on or around the body, the Chakra itself is not your physical body but a separate body of energy either within your own body. Meditating on the Chakra points is said to give you a greater awareness not only of yourself and the workings of your body but of the world around you, both physical and spiritual.

There are seven Chakra points, each corresponding to a different place on the body.

- The Sahasrara, or Crown, is the topmost of the Chakra and is located, as the name suggests, in the crown of your head. To meditate on Sahasrara is to meditate on the highest form of consciousness and self-realization.

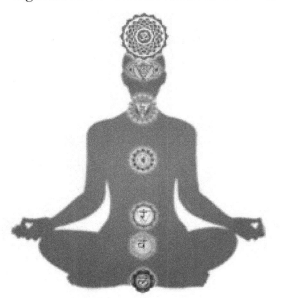

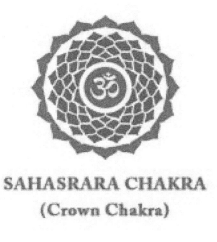

**SAHASRARA CHAKRA**
(Crown Chakra)

- The Ajna, or Third Eye, is located between the eyebrows. To meditate on Ajna is to     meditate on the union of opposites.

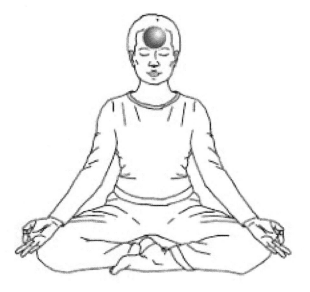

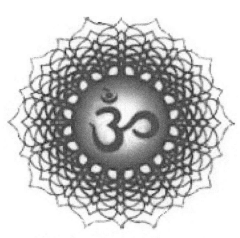

*Chakra 6 - chez Francesca*

- The Vishuddha, or Throat, is located, not surprisingly, in the throat. To meditate on Vishuddha is to meditate on creativity.

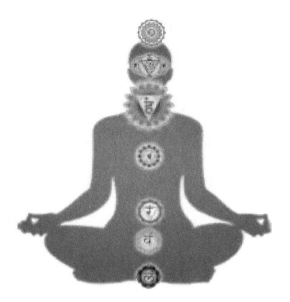 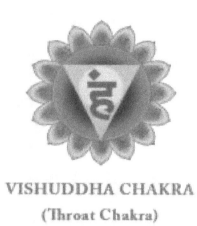

**VISHUDDHA CHAKRA**
(Throat Chakra)

- The Anahata, or Heart, it located in the heart. To meditate on Anahata is to meditate on balance.

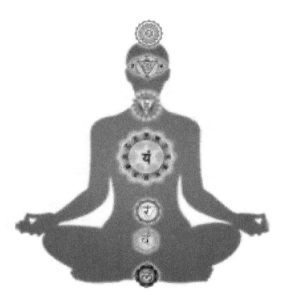 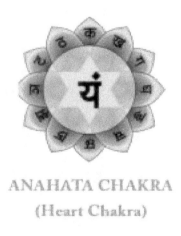

**ANAHATA CHAKRA**
(Heart Chakra)

- The Manipura, or Solar Plexus, is located in the navel. To meditate on Manipura is to meditate on creation and destruction.

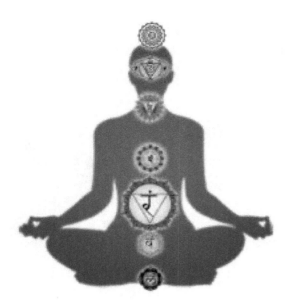

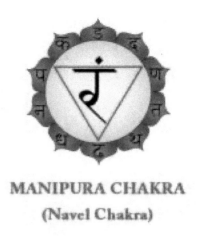

**MANIPURA CHAKRA**
**(Navel Chakra)**

- The Svadhishthana, or Sacral, is located at the base of the sexual organs. To meditate on Svadhishthana is to meditate on clarity.

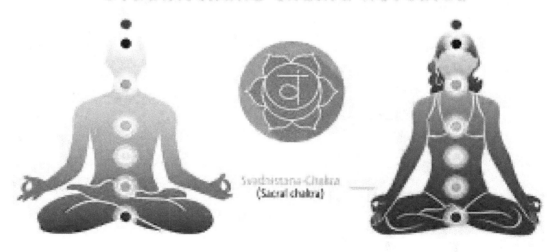

Svadhisthana Chakra Revealed

Svadhisthana-Chakra
(Sacral chakra)

- The Muladhara, or Root, is located at the base of the spine. To meditate on Muladhara is to meditate on Kundalini ('Coiled One'), or the energy that resides within your spine.

# The Secrets of Muladhara Chakra

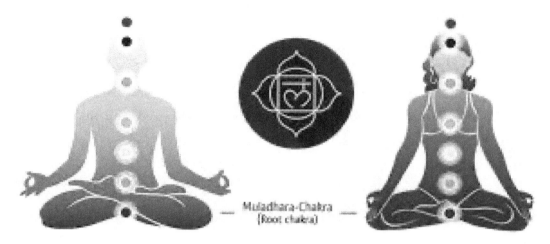

Muladhara-Chakra
(Root chakra)

Whichever method of Mindfulness Meditation you choose, remember that the goal is to unite with the world around you and become one with yourself.

# Chapter 10    Affirmation

Did you know that your brain operates with something that functions like a computer's operating system? Seriously. If you take two people and you teach them to think of themselves in two different ways, they would start acting differently. They both have the same hardware. They both have roughly the same physiology. What separates them is what they choose to believe about themselves.

Imagine having two computers in front of you. You can have the exact same hardware configuration, the same amount of memory, storage, and bandwidth speed. The only difference is on one computer you install an operating system that only allows you to use that computer as a word processor. On the other computer, you install an operating system that only permits spreadsheet operations. What do you think will happen?

It's not rocket science. On the computer with the word processing application, you obviously can only do word processing. The other computer is only capable of doing spreadsheets. The same applies to human beings.

Depending on our programming, we can only achieve a certain range of activities. If you are an unsuccessful person, or you feel that you could be earning more money or your net worth could be much higher, maybe it's because you chose to adopt a certain type of programming that prevented you from achieving the kind of success that you feel you deserve. If you have more a few extra pounds and have always wanted to adopt a 'healthier lifestyle' but can't seem to get around to it, maybe it's because of the programming you have chosen. Maybe you eat lots of sweet or greasy food for 'comfort.' Whatever you're trying to fix in your life, it can be traced to programming and affirmation meditation can help you achieve serious breakthroughs.

**It all boils down to what you wish to learn and unlearn**

Affirmation meditation is all about becoming conscious of this programming process, and taking active and deliberate control over it. It's very important to pay attention to the level of deliberation required.

The thing with most human beings is that we all operate under some sort of programming. Most of us were programmed by our parents. By simply being around them, we tend to pick up their habits and it doesn't take long for us to essentially act like their clones at a certain level. This is especially true when it comes to our values.

Your programming has to come from somewhere. Your programming doesn't just magically appear. You have picked them up from people or from circumstances. They are never random or 'come from within.' They are learned.

What's important to note is that not all of this is conscious. In fact, for most people, this is almost always unconscious or automatic because of their environment.

Affirmation meditation involves overriding your programming and consciously reprogramming yourself through a willful mantra. Unlike the mantra-based meditation practice it's a fully conscious process and you can either choose to do it with your eyes closed or you can do it in front of a mirror where you can see your image and talk to it.

## How it works

The first step to affirmation meditation is to pick empowering short statements. You have to be very careful regarding what these statements are because they program you to start thinking of yourself a certain way.

If you keep this up long enough, you start believing it and you start acting on it. That's how powerful they are. So they must have a specific meaning and specific depth. They cannot be shallow and simplistic. They have to engage your mind on many different levels.

One of the most common types of affirmation statements is "I am" statements. I call these power statements because the phrase "I am" is self-definition. When you say "I am," you tell the universe-and yourself-who you are. You define yourself. This is why it's very, very dangerous when people repeat certain "I am" statements in an almost unthinking, habitual way.

For example, how many times have you said to yourself whether silently or audibly that you're a loser, or you're broke and you don't have any money, or you're poor? When you do this, you're not just letting off steam. I wish it was that simple and innocent. Instead, when you say these statements, you're actually reprogramming your personal reality. That's why it's really important to be as conscious as possible and be very discriminating regarding the "I am" power statements you choose.

Personally, I have used "I am worthy," "I am faith," "I am trust," "I am love," "I am kind," and other related "I am" statements.

These are not random statements because they are very, very deep. They have very broad implications. When you say you are worthy, this means that you have a certain level of mastery. You can be trusted. You can be expected to lead people where they need to go. You also have certain capabilities. This is some deep stuff.

It's really important to pick your mental affirmation statement very, very carefully. It has to be meaningful and it has to be deep. It has to resonate because your mind is always listening and is extremely sensitive. What you choose to adopt for certain parts of your life-say money management or your health habits-can have consequences for other areas of your life. For example, if you have the habit of always saying 'I am broke' this can impact your ability to come up with solutions for other areas of your life.

By being conscious and deliberate regarding your power statements, you can override whatever faulty or negative programming your life maybe suffering from. One common example of this is your parents scolding you when you were a kid telling you that you're a bad kid, you're lazy, and you're no good. While it's easy to brush them off, those statements can leave a profound subconscious impact. Affirmation meditation is all about overriding those.

## The secret to success

To truly make affirmation meditation work for you, you have to pair it with breathing exercises and a relaxed state. By simply counting your breath and achieving a relaxed mental state before you issue power statements, you explode the power of your power statements. What you want to avoid is just simply saying an empty phrase over and over again. While it may produce substantive results later on, it's going to take much longer.

To really turbocharge the results that you can get from this meditation method, you have to pair it with breathing exercises and a deeply relaxed state of mind, you then zero in on your power statement and this can have a deep and profound impact on your mental, emotional, and physical state. You feel relaxed, but you also feel empowered.

I wish I could tell you that the affirmation method is quick and easy, but it isn't. It takes some practice. That's why I would suggest that you need to gain some familiarity with the other meditation techniques outlined in this book before you try this method out. The good news is that once you are able to reach a relaxed mental state of being and you have picked the right power statements, this method can help you reprogram your life very, very rapidly.

# Chapter 11    Tricks for Relieving Anxiety, Depression, and Insomnia

Most people feel unsure and stuck when they get anxious, not knowing what to do to turn their mood around. You may even unintentionally make your anxiety even stronger by obsessing about the future or ruminating about something that happened earlier in the day. You may ask yourself what could go wrong and run through endless scenarios, making yourself more upset with each passing thought. And worst of all, you may even bash yourself and judge your own thoughts and anxiety, believing in all the worst-case ideas you can come up with.

## How to Reduce Anxiety

But it doesn't have to be this way. You can change these patterns. There are many different techniques and tools you can implement to help curb your anxiety. Meditation is, of course, a great place to start, but there are other tricks you can use to make it even more effective. Let's look a little closer at these now.

### Deep Breathing

The best thing to do as soon as you start feeling anxious is to take a deep breath. There's a reason why this advice is so cliché and well-known; because it works! Deep breathing from the belly can reduce your anxiety because it automatically turns on the relaxation response in your body, soothing your nervous feelings. Inhale for four seconds, filling up your belly and chest, hold the breath for four seconds, and then exhale for four seconds. Repeat this until you feel better.

### Acceptance

The next crucial step is accepting where you are with your anxious thoughts. Anxiety is nothing but an emotion, just like any other. When you remind yourself that it's just a feeling reaction instead of an emergency, acceptance becomes much easier. Acceptance is a must because attempting to force yourself to stop feeling anxious just makes it worse, as you likely already know. It only feeds the false notion that anxiety is unacceptable or intolerable.

Contrary to what you may think, when you accept anxious feelings, you aren't giving up or accepting misery. Instead, you're being realistic and allowing yourself to let your emotions flow through and pass. All emotions will naturally pass on their own if you don't resist them. So next time, try acceptance!

## See the Illusion

When you're in a panicked frenzy of anxious thoughts, your brain is messing with you. Realizing this can help you combat anxiety. A panic attack can actually feel like a severe health issue, but it isn't. You will not die from anxiety, even if it feels like you might at any moment, and it pays to remind yourself of this.

## Question Reality

Anytime someone gets anxious, their minds begin throwing outlandish ideas at them. No matter how unlikely or unrealistic these ideas are, the anxious mind will latch onto them and feed them with fear. Next time these thoughts start to run through your head, try questioning them instead. Say you're about to give a presentation at work and immediately think, "I cannot do this, I'm going to fail and embarrass myself." Instead of instantly believing the thought and letting it grow in intensity, remind yourself that the situation isn't an emergency and that you've survived fear before.

But when we're anxious, we often perceive events as worse than they really are. Even if you do mess up on your presentation, the people in the audience will be so concerned with their own thoughts that they will probably hardly notice. Here are some questions you can ask yourself next time you feel anxious:

- Am I being realistic right now?

- 

- What is the likeliest outcome of this event?

- 

- Can I handle it if things go wrong?

- 
  - What can I do to help this situation?
- 
  - Is there a way to prepare that I haven't thought of yet?
- 
  - Am I getting carried away with fear right now?

**Learn How to Visualize**

Practice this meditation on a regular basis, and it will help you gain access to peace next time you're feeling nervous. Imagine that you're next to a lake or river at your favorite place. Feel the sun on your face, hear the water, and sense your calm state of mind. Imagine that each cloud floating by is one of your emotions, and allow them to pass. Emotions are not inherently good or bad. They are neutral, and we assign labels to them. But you don't have to do this. Remember that every feeling is neutral and that you can choose how to handle it.

**Observe with No Judgment**

One of the main goals of your meditation can be observing your judgment, sensations, feelings, and thoughts with a compassionate attitude instead of the judgment you would usually have. Write this goal down and keep it somewhere highly visible so you can be reminded of what it says.

**Using Positive Words**

Most of us aren't very mindful of how we speak to ourselves, and that just makes anxiety worse. Instead of allowing yourself to engage in hateful, self-destructive talk in your head, focus instead on positive words. Remind yourself that you are strong, capable, and worthy of love.

**Be Present-focused**

Anxiety can only exist when you are projecting yourself into the past or future. When you're present in the hear and now, it goes away. Next time you're obsessing about something that already happened or will happen, remember that you can't control anything other than your attitude in the present moment. Take some deep breaths, do a short meditation, and return to the situation with new eyes.

**Stay Busy**

Any time you're feeling anxious, it can be hard to accomplish the tasks that you normally would throughout the day, but this is exactly what you should do. Instead of sitting down and obsessing, avoiding your tasks, or distracting yourself, go about your to-do list as if it were just an ordinary day. Be busy, and your anxious feelings will fade naturally as all emotions do.

## Tricks for Relieving Depression

Depression is a difficult matter to deal with, but a few of these tips can help you manage it better. Although meditation can help with depression, don't neglect seeing a mental health professional if you feel it isn't enough. Here are the tips:

### 1. Be Smart about Your Goals

Choose some straightforward, easy goals that you can follow without much issue. They should be measurable, specific, rewarding, and possible. In other words, choosing that you will lose 20 pounds within a week isn't a realistic goal, but choosing to go for a walk each day is.

### 2. Avoid Dramatic Thinking

Thinking in black and white terms feeds depression. People who are feeling depressed tend to think that no one likes them or that they'll never amount to anything. This type of dramatic thinking just makes depression worse. Meditation can help a lot with separating yourself from these thoughts, but you can also try thinking in gray shades instead of black and white. Instead of using language such as "always" or "never," ask yourself how realistic you're being and find a statement that more accurately reflects reality. For example, if you think "I'll never get a job," immediately replace it with, "I will find a job because I have done so many times in the past."

**Fake it till you Make It**

When you're depressed, you will probably stop doing the activities that you care about most in the world. Make a list of these activities, such as taking walks, seeing friends, or cooking at home. Even if you don't feel like it, start reintroducing each of these activities into your schedule. Odds are, once you begin following through with them, some of your enthusiasm will return, and you'll feel better. Even taking care of errands can make you feel better than sitting around and doing nothing.

**Look for Evidence**

Depressive thoughts are rarely realistic. Next time you feel depressed, remember that your thoughts are likely colored by the mental state and aren't based on evidence. As soon as a negative thought comes up, ask to see the evidence of it. Odds are, you won't find any evidence for the belief that "Everyone hates me." Decide to stop repeating these harmful ideas to yourself, and never assume you know what others think of you unless you've asked.

**Accept the Mental State**

The worst thing you can do when you feel depressed is deny it. If your situation sucks at the moment, just accept where you are. That's the only way you can move past it. Acceptance is the only way to relieve your state of suffering because it opens up your mind to see solutions.

**Be Nice to Yourself**

Treating yourself with respect is another important foundation for a healthy mentality in life. Pay attention to how you speak to yourself compared to how you talk to other people. If you're way meaner to yourself than you are to others (which you likely are in this case), make an effort to be gentler and kinder in your self-talk. Think about whether you'd use the same words you talk to yourself with while comforting your best friend. If not, the language has no place in your mind.

**Find Structure**

Even when you aren't in the mood, always follow a schedule of some kind. Set your alarm for the morning, eat lunch at the same time, and go to sleep around the same time, as well. When you're depressed, it's easy to fall into habits of sleeping or eating inconsistently. Even when you're feeling down or are unemployed, setting a structured routine is important as it can give you a reliable setting to focus on. Bonus points if you can fit socializing into the routine.

## Tricks to Relieve Sleeplessness

What is insomnia? It's being unable to either fall or stay asleep, which results in non-restorative and unrefreshing rest at night. Everyone needs different amounts of rest at night, so insomnia can be defined as how you feel after waking up instead of how fast you can fall asleep or the amount of hours you stay asleep. Even for those who lie down for eight hours every night, waking up feeling fatigued and drowsy could still mean they have insomnia.

When it comes to sleep complaints, insomnia is the most common, but it doesn't refer to just one sleep disorder. It makes more sense to call it a symptom of a problem than the problem itself. Whatever issue is causing sleeplessness will be different between individuals. It could be that you have a medical condition or that you've simply had too much coffee that day.

### Symptoms of Insomnia

Thankfully, most insomnia can be fixed by making personal changes without sleeping pills or visiting a professional. Let's look at some common symptoms of insomnia:

- Being tired but still having trouble falling asleep

-

- Waking up a lot throughout the night

-

- Not being able to fall asleep again after waking up

-

- Waking up in the morning still very tired

-

- Needing alcohol or drugs to get to sleep at night

- 
- Waking up earlier than you want to repeatedly
- 
- Being irritable, tired, or drowsy during the day
- 
- Having a hard time concentrating due to tiredness

## Potential Causes

To be able to cure or treat your sleeplessness, you have to start paying attention. This is where meditation can be a great help. Emotional problems like depression or anxiety are the cause of at least 50 percent of cases of insomnia. But the habits you have during the day and before sleeping can also play a part in sleeplessness. In addition, your physical habits play a role. Try to indicate all potential causes of sleeplessness, and as soon as you've found a root issue, you can work on treating it. Here are some potential causes of insomnia:

- Are you going through something stressful in your life?
- 
- Do you feel hopeless, flat, or depressed?
- 
- Have you experienced trauma recently?
- 
- Are you suffering from constant worry or anxiety?
- 
- Did you recently start any new medications?
- 
- Is there a health issue that might be causing the issue?

- 

- Is your bedroom comfortable and quiet for sleeping?

- 

- Do you have a consistent schedule of sleeping and waking?

## Medical or Psychological Causes

At times, sleeplessness will only last a couple days and then goes away. This is especially true when it's from a temporary cause like jet lag, a breakup, or a presentation that's making you feel nervous. But other times, it sticks around. This is when it could be related to a physical or mental issue that you have yet to identify. Let's look at a list of medical or psychological causes for insomnia, some of which may require treatment from a professional:

- Anxiety disorder or recurring stress

- 

- Depression or consistent sadness

- 

- Persistent anger and frustration

- 

- Trauma, grief, or bipolar disorder

- 

- Asthma or allergies

- 

- Acid reflux from diet problems

- 

- Kidney issues

-

- Chronic pain

-

- Parkinson's disease

## Sleep Disorders

Persistent insomnia is a sleep disorder itself, but may also signify a different sleep disorder like restless legs syndrome, sleep apnea, or disturbances in your circadian rhythm due to odd work hours or traveling.

## Medications

Certain medications can cause sleeplessness, like some contraceptives, blood pressure meds, thyroid hormones, ADHD stimulants, and antidepressant medications. Flue and cold meditations might cause sleeplessness if they have alcohol in them. Diuretics, Model, Excedrin, and diet pills can also cause insomnia as they often have caffeine or other stimulants in them.

## How to Figure Out the Cause

Although treating mental and underlying physical issues is good to start with, it won't always take away your insomnia completely. You should also take a look at the habits you engage in during the day as your coping methods for sleeplessness may actually contribute to the problem, in some cases. For instance, you might be relying on alcohol or sleeping pills to go to sleep at night, which only contributes to the issue over time. Or you might be drinking too much coffee at work, keeping you up at night. Here are some other habits that could contribute:

- Taking naps during the day

-

- Having too much sugar during the day

-

- Eating too much at night

- 
- Exercising late in the day
- 
- Not moving around enough
- 
- Using your phone before bed
- 
- Watching movies before sleep

These habits not only make insomnia worse but sleeping badly can make you rely on these habits even more, creating an unhealthy cycle. The only way to break out of this cycle is to change the habits contributing to it. At times, these simple changes will be enough to get rid of the insomnia issue. Give yourself a few days to get accustomed to this change, but as soon as you do, it could solve the problem. Don't forget to look at habits that you may not typically associate with sleep problems. Some habits might be so automatic that you don't realize they can be a factor. You might have to give up your nightly glass of wine or phone habit before bed.

# Chapter 12    What is Self-Hypnosis?

Self-hypnosis is still considered a mystical phenomenon by many people, even though this technique can be seen as prayer. You are alone and you concentrate on your well-being. If you like, you ask God or a supreme being you believe in to help you. This practice also includes meditation (just like praying does), as well as chanting, mantras, inner confirmation or affirmation. When you have to perform at work or at college, you make such statements like "I don't fear; I'm fine"; "I can do it" or exactly the opposite like "I can't do it. Everybody is better than me", etc. Even when we imagine ourselves in a different scenario from what is currently happening, we are programming ourselves. What you are doing is continuously hypnotizing yourself. Self-hypnosis helps us to come into contact with the unconscious through the use of a specific language, aimed at awakening some parts of ourselves by leveraging archetypal symbols. Self-hypnotization is self-programming. Our unconscious understands the symbolic messages of words rather than their rational meaning; that's why figurative language is used in hypnosis for inducing the individual to relax and to focus on the inner world. We are embedding a vivid, information-rich image with emotions in the subconscious mind.

However, we must learn to pray or let's say hypnotize ourselves accurately! Self-hypnosis is the ability to apply techniques and procedures alone to stimulate the unconscious to become our ally and involve it directly in the realization of our goals. By learning the essential elements of communication with the unconscious mind, it is possible to become able to reprogram activities of our unconscious. Self-hypnosis is a method that does not dismiss the support of a professional but has the advantage of being able to be performed independently. This is possible through the use of CDs and DIY courses made by hypnotists to make this practice accessible to a larger number of people with significant advantages, even from an economic point of view!

**What is self-hypnosis for?**

It was Milton H. Erickson, founder of modern hypnotherapy, who gave an exhaustive illustration of the effects and purposes of hypnosis and self-hypnosis. The scholar stated that the aim of this practice is to communicate with the subconscious of the subjects through the use of metaphors and stories full of symbolic meanings (Tyrrell, 2014).

If incorrectly applied, self-hypnosis can certainly not harm, but it may not be useful in attaining the desired results, with the risk of not feeling motivated to continue a constructive relationship with the unconscious. However, to do it as efficiently as possible, we need to be in a relaxed state of mind. So, accordingly, we start with relaxation to gather the attention inside, while suspending conscious control. Then we insert suggestions and affirmations to the unconscious mind. At the end of the time allocated for the process, a gradual awakening procedure facilitates the return to the state of permanent consciousness. When you are calm, your subconscious is 20-25% more programmable than when you are agitated. Also, it effectively relieves stress (you can repair a lot of information and stimuli you understand), aids regeneration, energizes, triggers positive physiological changes, improves concentration, helps you find solutions, and helps you make the right decisions. If the state of conscious trance is reached, then if the patient manages to let himself go by concentrating on the words of the hypnotist, progressively forgetting the external stimuli, then the physiological parameters undergo considerable variations. The confirmation comes from science, and in fact, it was found that during hypnosis, the left hemisphere, the rational one, decreases its activity in favor of the more creative hemisphere, the right one (Harris, n. d.).

You can do self-hypnosis in faster and more immediate ways, even during the course of the various daily activities after you have experienced what state you need to reach during hypnosis.

A better understanding of communication with the unconscious mind highlights how indispensable our collaboration is to slip into the state outside the ordinary consciousness. In other words, we enter an altered state of consciousness because we want it, and every form of hypnosis, even if induced by someone else, is always self-hypnosis.

We wish to access the extraordinary power of unconscious creativity; for this, we understand that it is necessary to put aside for a while the control of the rational mind and let ourselves slip entirely into relaxation and into the magical world of the unconscious where everything is possible.

Immense benefits can be obtained from a relationship that becomes natural and habitual with one's own unconscious. Self-hypnosis favors the emergence of constructive responses from our being, can allow us to know ourselves better, helps us to be more aware of our potential, and more able to express them and use them to foster our success in every field of possible application.

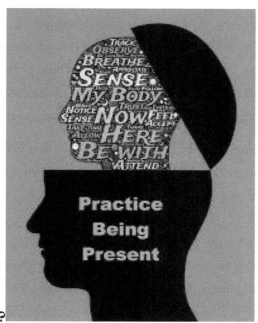

**How do you do self-hypnosis?**

There are several self-hypnosis techniques out there; however, they are all based on one concept: focusing on a single idea, object, image, or word. This is the key that opens the door to trance. You can achieve focus in many ways, which is the reason why there are so many different techniques that can be applied. After a period of initial learning, those who have learned a method, and have continued to practice it, realize that they can skip certain steps. In this part, we will take a look at the essential self-hypnosis techniques.

The Betty Erickson Method

Here I'll summarize the most practical points of this method of Betty Erickson, wife of Milton Erickson, the most famous hypnotist of 1900.

Choose something you don't like about yourself. Turn it into an image, and then turn this image into a positive one. If you don't like your body shape, take a picture of your body, then turn it into an image of your beautiful self with a body you would like to have. Before inducing self-hypnosis, give yourself a time limit before hypnotizing yourself by mentally or better yet, saying aloud the following sentence, "I induce self-hypnosis for X minutes". Your mind will take time like a Swiss watch.

**How do you practice?**

Take three objects around you, preferably small and bright, like a door handle, a light spot on a painting, etc. and fix your attention on each one of them. Take three sounds from your environment, traffic, fridge noise, etc., and fix your attention on each one. Take three sensations you are feeling, the itchy nose, tingling in the leg, the feeling of air passing through the nose, etc. It's better to use unusual sensations, to which attention is not usually drawn, such as the sensation of the right foot inside the shoe. Don't fix your attention for too long, just enough to make you aware of what you are seeing, feeling or trying. The mind is quick. Then, in the same way, switch to two objects, two sounds, two sensations. Always be calm, while switching to an object, a sound, a sensation. If you have done things correctly, you are in a trance, ready for the next step.

Now let your mind wander, as you did in class, when the teacher spoke and you looked out of the window, and you were in another place, in another time, in another space, in a place where you would have liked to be, so completely forget about everything else. Now recall the initial image. Perhaps the mind wanders, from time to time it gets distracted, maybe it goes adrift, but it doesn't matter. As soon as you can, take the initial image, and start working on it. Do not make efforts to try to remind you of what it means or what it is. Your mind works according to mental associations, let it work at its best without unnecessarily disturbing it: it knows what it must do. Manipulate the image, play with it a little. See if it looks brighter, or if it is smaller, or it is more pleasant. If it is a moving image, send it back and forth in slow motion or speed it up. When the initial image always gets worse, replace it instantly with the second image.

Reorientation, also known as awakening, marks the end of self-hypnotic induction. Enjoy your new image, savor it as much as you like, and when you have done this, open your eyes. If you have not given yourself any time limits before entering self-hypnosis, when you are satisfied with the work done, count quietly to yourself from one to ten and wake up, and open your eyes (Traversa, 2018).

The Benson Method

Herbert Benson, in his famous book titled, *Relaxation Response,* describes the methods and results of some tests carried out on a group of meditators dedicated to "transcendental meditation" to reach concentration (1975). Benson suggested a method of relaxation based on the concentration of the mind on a single idea which was incorporated in the Eastern disciplines. The technique includes the following steps:

- Meditate on one word, but you can choose an object or something else if you want to.

- Sit down in a quiet place and close your eyes. Relax the muscles and direct attention to the breath.

- Think silently about the object of meditation and continue to do so for 10-20 minutes. If you find that you have lost the object of meditation, gather your focus again on the original object.

- Once the set time is reached, open your eyes stretch yourself well for some additional minutes. Obviously, to perform better, you will need to practice.

Benson proposes this exercise as a meditation practice. In reality, there are no differences between the hypnotic state and that achieved with meditation. This is one of the most straightforward self-hypnosis exercises you can do.

Here is another simple technique that was developed by the first hypnotists because it leads to a satisfactory state of trance in a reasonable time. It can be used to enter self-hypnosis in a short time.

- Sit down in a quiet place and close your eyes. Relax the muscles and direct attention to the breath.

- Begin to open and close your eyes by counting slowly. Open your eyes at the odd numbers close them at the even numbers. Continue counting very slowly and slowing down the numbering of even numbers.

- After a few numbers, your eyes become tired, and you find it difficult to open them at odd numbers. Continue counting while you can open your eyes at the odd numbers. If you cannot do it, it means you are in a trance.

- Go deeper by slowly counting twenty other numbers. Let yourself go to the images, to the sensations, and to the words that come to mind. To wake up from the trance, count from one to five, and open your eyes at five (Stress Management Plus, n. d.).

These are examples of techniques, but no one is preventing you from devising others, as long as the underlying assumption is maintained: concentration on a single idea.

# Conclusion

Thank you for making it through to the end of Guide Meditation for Anxiety and Insomnia, let's hope it was informative and able to provide you with all of the tools you need to achieve your goals whatever they may be.

The next step is to take what you read and apply it to the moments that you feel is making you the most anxious or on the brink of a panic attack or for situations, that you feel could cause an event.

With many people experiencing a high amount of anxiety today, there is not a lot of information leading up to the actual prevention of anxiety or true treatment options from a medical point of view. That is why this book is jam-packed with various ways that can either relieve or eliminate the signs and symptoms associated with anxiety by way of self-guided meditations.

As you read, you will now be able to calm yourself in a much faster amount of time and before your anxiety can get out of control and become a full-blown panic attack.

CPSIA information can be obtained
at www.ICGtesting.com
Printed in the USA
LVHW101932190121
676908LV00009B/264